VAGUS NERVE

How the Vagus Nerve Can Help Combat Anxiety

(How to Activate Your Healing Power the Secrets
to Eliminate Stress and Depression)

Steven Kaster

Published By Harry Barnes

Steven Kaster

All Rights Reserved

Vagus Nerve: How the Vagus Nerve Can Help Combat Anxiety (How to Activate Your Healing Power the Secrets to Eliminate Stress and Depression)

ISBN 978-1-77485-261-3

Legal & Disclaimer

The information contained in this book is not designed to replace or take the place of any form of medicine or professional medical advice. The information in this book has been provided for educational and entertainment purposes only.

The information contained in this book has been compiled from sources deemed reliable, and it is accurate to the best of the Author's knowledge; however, the Author cannot guarantee its accuracy and validity and cannot be held liable for any errors or omissions. Changes are periodically made to this book. You must consult your doctor or get professional medical advice before using any of the suggested remedies, techniques, or information in this book.

Upon using the information contained in this book, you agree to hold harmless the Author from and against any damages, costs, and expenses, including any legal fees potentially resulting from the application of any of the information provided by this guide. This disclaimer applies to any damages or injury caused by the use and application, whether directly or indirectly, of any advice or information presented, whether for breach of contract, tort, negligence, personal injury, criminal intent, or under any other cause of action.

You agree to accept all risks of using the information presented inside this book. You need to consult a professional medical practitioner in order to ensure you are both able and healthy enough to participate in this program.

Table of Contents

Introduction

The nerve that controls vagus. It's not a subject that's taught in the classroom or in our lives yet it's incredibly vital for the health and wellbeing that our body.

It's a nerve that is located in our brains that a lot of us aren't aware about. However, the vagus nerve plays an important part in the occurrence of problems within the body, as well as aids in the correction of existing problems.

We don't be aware of this brain nerve. So, this book is precisely the information you need to know more about this nerve. The book is going to discuss more about vagus muscle, as well as the function it plays and the reason why it's crucial.

The reality is that the vagus nerve is involved in far more than we imagine. It's a tiny collection of nerves and despite being to be the longest nerve in the body, it's not considered to be so by most people.

This book will explain everything you must learn about vagus nerve stimulation. We will discuss the reasons behind it what it is, why it's important and how stimulating this nerve may be the key for resolving many issues you are having.

Chapter 1: The Autonomic Nervous Systems

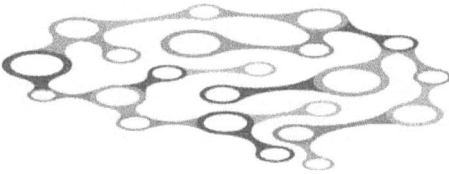

Autonomic nerves are a component of the nerve system. It manages the functions of internal organs. It is performed automatically, without effort, thinking or conscious consciousness of the individual. There are two major parts of the autonomic nerve system which are the sympathetic nervous system as well as parasympathetic system. Together both systems control external organs, glands as well as smooth muscle. There is a third system in the autonomic nerve system, called the enteric system.

Figure 1 Free Image

Three Systems of the Autonomic Nervous System Three Systems of the Autonomic Nervous System

The Sympathetic Nervous System. This section of the nerve system controls homeostasis or the balance of physiological functions, between the organs of the body. If it is activated consistently the basal level is maintained, which results in the process of maintaining homeostasis.

The neurons, from which are the ones that sympathetic nerve system works off, are located within the peripheral nerve system as well as in the spinal column that is part of the central nerve. They allow communication between the central sympathetic neuron to the sympathetic ganglia. They they are responsible for activating an increase in noradrenaline as well as adrenaline. This triggers or is connected in the body's fight fight response. In the event of this activation there are a variety of physiological changes occur in the body . These include:

* Changes in heart rate

* Open the airways

* Large intestine movement

* Pupil dilation

* Perspiration.

The sympathetic nerves may be situated in the middle of the inner side of vertebral column, and are disperse in the lateral Horn. They begin to protrude from the thoracic region the spinal cord, and extend out into the third and second lumbar regions. The nerve fibers, or axons are pushed out of the spinal column to ventral branches, and connect to the chain ganglia on the right and left sides of vertebral columns. Through these connections, connections are created which allow nerves to reach glands, organs, and other parts of the body.

If you are confronted with an intimidating or stressful situation the nervous system of sympathetic nerves is put into high alert and activates an instinctual response of fight and flight. The result is several reactive reactions that range from anger to withdrawal or even withdrawal.

The parasympathetic nerve system. While the sympathetic nervous system responds rapidly when stimulated, the parasympathetic nervous system is slower to activate. The parasympathetic system is situated within the area between the spine and brain. It plays a role in the correct function of glands as well as organs. This includes:

* The heart rate is slowed down

* Relieving the muscles

* Sexual arousal

* Tear production

* Salivation

* Digestion

* Urination

* Defecation.

The parasympathetic system is responsible to the digest and rest phases. This is opposed to the fight or flight response.

The enteric nervous system. The enteric system is situated in the middle of the body, or what is known as the solar system. It controls signals to the brain , and is able to perform autonomic functions. The majority of signals coming from the neuron 10 of the cranial nerve travel into the system of enteric nerves. The cranial nerve 10, also known as the vagus nerve makes communications between the nervous system of the enteric the central nervous system and sympathetic nerve system.

The link between the nerve fibers of the system, the cranial nerves and spinal nerves permits information to travel from one region of the body and then to the brain. This information is then transmitted to other parts of the body and triggers reactions triggered by external and internal influences.

The twelve Cranial Nerves

2. Free image

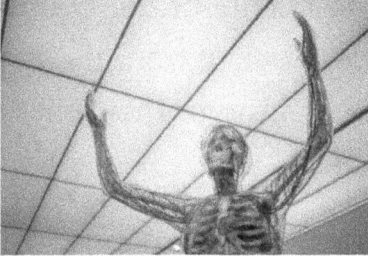

The Cranial nerves regulate sensory or motor functions within the body. Some of these nerves also fulfill both functions. They originate directly from the brain stem, and are component of the peripheral nerve system. It is the peripheral nerve system that is made up of ganglia and nerves that are not located directly within the the spinal column but are situated outside these regions. They are the 12 neuronal nerves of the cranium. are commonly called roman numerals ranging from 1-12, also known as I-XII. They are classified according to the location they originate out from the brain stem starting from beginning, which is through the middle of the brainstem and the last one, coming from the rear to the back of the brainstem. They are:

Olfactory- It is the primary cranial nerve. It is among the nerves that emerge from the forebrain or cerebrum rather than directly coming out of the stems of brain. Although this nerve is thought of as to be one of the peripheral nerve system, this nerve is commonly connected to the central nervous system. It is among the only cranial nerves which has the ability to renew itself. It is responsible for smell sensations.

Optic- Similar to the olfactory or olfactory nerve, the optic nerve is a part of the cerebrum. The optic nerve is the second one which is responsible for transmitting information about the visual system from the eye retina into the brain.

Oculomotor- This nerve is responsible for eye movements. It is able to constrict pupils, and it also controls eyelid movements, such as keeping the lid open.

The Trochlear nerve assists in eye movement specifically, such as the rotation of the eye. It is classified as motor nerve since it is connected to the superior Oblique muscles.

Trigeminal - The fifth cranial nerve regulates the functions of mouth and facial. It also senses the sensations of the mouth and face.

Abducens- It is a different motor nerve which connects the muscles of the lateral rectus region in the eyes. The nerve is responsible for controlling the lateral movement.

Facial nerve is responsible for muscle movements that transmit facial expressions. It also conveys sensations of taste along with functions associated with the front third of tongue as well as the oral cavity.

Vestibulocochlear This vestibulocochlear nerve is the one responsible for vestibular functions and for ensuring balance. It transmits audio or sound sensations from the ear's inner part and the brain.

The Glossopharyngeal nerve is the main receiver of signalling from the tonsils the pharynx, middle ear, and tongue.

Vagus is among the most complex nerves that regulates many functions in the body. It is connected to the brainstem to the abdomen. It's what makes breathing, speaking and muscle movements possible. It also regulates the heart rate, intestinal peristalsis, as well as sweating. The nerve will be discussed more thoroughly in the following chapter. Due to its length and the impact it has on various body functions and movements it is an important nerve to in reducing, eliminating or treat a variety of health conditions.

Spinal AccessoryThe 11th cervical nerve is responsible for controlling the muscles in the neck and shoulders.

Hypoglossal- The cranial nerve is focused on muscle movements that are connected with swallowing, speech, and chewing.

Treatment of the Cranial Nerves

Damage to the cranial nerves can happen because of tumors, injuries inflammation, trauma infection, insufficient blood supply and exposure to toxin. A single or a number of nerves in the cranium can be damaged and cause interference with the parts of the body that nerves regulate. Nerves may also malfunction or be damaged when specific parts of the brain which control the nerves get damaged. Common symptoms that can are experienced when there is a damage to the cranial nerve are:

* Facial pain that is intense and occurs and then disappears

* Vertigo, dizziness, or dizziness.

• Hearing loss or difficulty hearing loss

* Muscle weakness

* Muscles are paralyzed

* Unknown facial twitches.

Damage to the cranial nerves can heal itself over time. Only one cranial nerve able to regenerate itself is the cranial nerve 1, the one that is known as the olfactory nerve. It is possible to treat infections, or to reduce inflammation that can cause nerve injury. The surgical procedure may be required to alleviate symptoms related to certain nerve conditions. The stimulation of nerves can be done to strengthen and stimulate the cerebral nerves.

The Spinal Nerves

The spinal nerves originate out from the spinal cord. They form a major part of the peripheral nerve system, but they also make contact to central nerves. The spinal nerves are located on every one side of vertebral columns making up a total of 31 pairs. They are named in accordance with the vertebra they originate from. These spinal nerves get identified in accordance with the place they are the closest to within the body. From the total of 31 pairs, 8 are in the cervical spine twelve are in the thoracic region as well as five in the area of the lumbar region and five in the sacral region, and one is located in the coccygeal region. The nerves play a role in communicating between spinal cords and organs. They transmit sensory, motor autonomic and sensory signals. the nerves are known as mixed nerves. The spinal nerves consist of a sensory or dorsal root as well as a ventral motor root.

Figure 3. Free Image

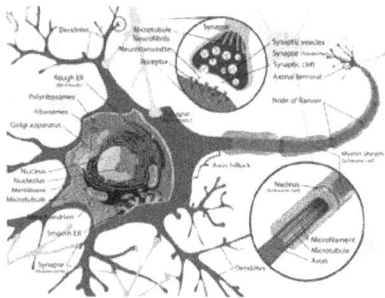

Your Body Is All Connected

The mind-body connection is characterized by clear communication from the body communicating data to the brain and processing messages returned to the body's organs to perform actions. The connection is a vital link between hormones, nerves, and neurotransmitters that trigger autonomous and involuntary reactions. It is based on the knowledge that our thoughts, emotions and experiences affect the body's capacity to function normally.

An excellent example of the connection between mind and body occurs when you experience feeling butterflies inside your stomach certain situations. This feeling of fluttering is your body's reaction to the feelings or thoughts the brain is processing. The brain connects to the major organs such as the lungs, heart and the digestive tract via the cranial nerves. It's not surprising that the way that you feel and how you perceive of the environment has an effect on the other parts part of the body. The strength of this connection is due to the neurotransmitters, chemicals, and hormones that the brain communicates the release and production of during different emotions. The hormones and chemicals are usually produced in different organs, such as the digestive tract as well as glands.

A strong connection between the mind and body is a sign of overall well-being. While all among the brain as well as spinal nerves perform specific functions and responsibilities to control the particular functions of the body The vagus nerve is the one with an even greater range of influence.

Chapter 2: The Vagus Nerve What Is It? Where Is It?

Our bodies are very complex, and our brains and our central nervous system that it manages are extremely complicated. In this case the goal of this chapter is to examine the 12 nerves in the cranial system, to briefly explain their functions and to focus on the vagus nerve.

From the Brain and Brainstem The 12 Cranial Nerves We Have

The most vital parts of the central nervous system can be controlled and influenced by nerves coming from the bottom of the brain as well as the adjacent brainstem, that connects the brain with the spinal cord. Nerves also come out of the spinal cord. The 12 nerves higher than the spine and are limited only to brainstem and its underlying structures are referred to as the cranial nerves. Each cranial nerve is a dual nerve that connects to both side of the brain as well as the brainstem. They are classified by their Roman numerals I through XII. These numbers correspond to the order in which every cranial nerve connectedto, which means that I is the most ahead, while XII is the last one in the brainstem. It is situated just above the highest point of the spinal column.

Knowing the role that each of the cranial nerves requires some practice However, for us the following descriptions will give you a solid foundation:

Olfactory is the nerve responsible to sense smell. It is able to repair or regenerate itself when damaged, an ability that very few nerves possess. They connect the brain (not the brainstem) to a variety of olfactory receptors within the nasal cavity.

Optic is the nerve that lets us see, through the retina that is located to the back of the eye to the portion of the brain which converts electrical impulses into the vision. The optic nerves form part of our central nervous system, and are the only neuron in the cranial region that is not connected to brainstem.

Oculomotor is the nerve that controls movements of the eye in opening up the lid, as well as allowing the pupil to constrict and dilate.

Trochlear is motor nerve that regulates the muscles which allow the eyeball to turn.

Trigeminal nerve, which has both sensory and motor functions that affect the face and mouth.

Abducens is another motor nerve that allows eye movements; here it's used for lateral motion.

Facial, another nerve which has sensation and motor functions. It enables us to use facial expressions, as well as tasting sensations emanating from the front two-thirds mouth and tongue.

Vestibulocochlear This nerve performs two functions: transmission of sound and equilibrium (equilibrium) signals to brain, originating from its origins within the inner auditory canal.

The Glossopharyngeal nerve is responsible for sensing information coming from the back of the tonsils and tongue and also from the larynx as well as the pharynx. There are also the sensations that emanate from the middle ear.

Vagus, a multi-tasking nerve is one out of all the 12 nerves in the cranial system that is responsible for heart rate and peristalsis (the contraction of the gastrointestinal system in order to transport food) and the operation of sweat glands. It also regulates speech and mouth movements. it regulates breathing by keeping the larynx open.

Spinal Accessory is the nerve that allows muscles in the shoulders and neck to perform their functions.

Hypoglossal is the brain nerve that controls tongue movements, including swallowing and manipulating food. It also allows speech.

The framework is now in place lets us concentrate solely on the X. the vagus nerve to comprehend and appreciate its variety of essential tasks.

The Tenth Longest and Tenth The Longest Cranial Nerve

Since there are twelve cranial nerves and the vagus nerve is one of them, it does not "do everything." However, it does a good job. In general, it's an important player and facilitator for your central nervous system. As you've seen the vagus nerve involved in the control of important areas of our heads which includes our mouth and throat. It also controls important aspects of digestion as well as the abdomen region. It also affects the lungs and thus our breathing. If all that is not enough, it has a direct impact on the majority of our vital organs and functions the vagus nerve directly responsible for the heart rate once it is at the top of the heart, where it triggers the sinoatrial node activating the beating impulses which shut and open the left and right atria. This allows blood to flow through and be delivered to ventricles. This means that the vagus nerve directly influences the rate of heart beat and blood pressure , and may cause increases or decreases of each.

To ensure that you get all recognition to the "great multitasker" vagus nerve is recognized as an information system that provides feedback to the brain know the condition of various organs of the body, and in particular the viscera. It encompasses all parts that comprise the digestive tract. These include the stomach, the esophagus as well as the large and small intestinal tracts.

We'll be more specific in the next chapter about the autonomic nervous systems and its sympathetic and parasympathetic system (both of which are influenced by the vagus nerve) However, for this moment, let's examine the way that our wanderer's nerve wanders.

Head To Gut Head To Gut Wandering Vagus Nerve

As a double nerve as with the other 12 cranial nerves, it has two pathways to follow that both descend into the brain, and the brainstem. The right and left vagus nerves descend from the brainstem into the carotid sheath. They are in a parallel or lateral direction with the carotidartery. The right vagus nerve descends to on the left side of the throat while the left vagus nerve runs the same way for the other side. running along the jugular vein and finally down between the jugular artery and the carotid arterial. Both sides continue to descend to the chest, where distinct nerve fibers branch, like they do into the abdomen region. The vagus nerve ultimately affects motor functions that influence the heart, lungs, bronchi , and the digestive tract. It also influences the sensory functions within the same organs along with the larynx and pharynx when it enters the neck.

The most effective way to comprehend the vagus nerve's proliferative network is to imagine an ongoing branching reaching across various organs, as the vagus nerve extends from the brainstem, into to the neck (where it connects to the larynx and pharynx) then out to connect to the lungs and heart before branching out to connect with various parts in the digestive system from the upper esophagus into the colon.

Chapter 3: What's The Vagus Nerve, And What Are Its Purposes

The strength to control the Vagus nerve. Vagus nerve is a powerful source of power. Vagus nerve is commonly referred to as the pneumogastric nervous system and can be described as the 10th nerve , or CNX and connects to the parasympathetic administration of the lungs, the heart as well as the digestion system. It is believed that the Vagus nerves are typically called in the singular. This is by far the most long nerve that exists in the human body, and an independent device. The terminal stage of Vagus nerve is regarded as the trigeminal nerve of the spinal cord.

Its roots are on the medulla Oblongata (also called the marrow oblongata).It connects the olivary nucleus as well as the cerebellar peduncles that are inferior. Vagus nerve is affixed to the jugular foramen and through the carotid sheath, between the carotid artery inside as well as the internal jugular vein beneath the chest, neck and the abdomen. It helps in the security of the viscera reaching all the way to the colon. Apart from providing some output to several organs as well, the Vagus nerve typically contains between the majority of Afferent nerves, which provide sensory information about the central nervous system's body parts. The left and right Vagus nerves exit from the vault of the cranial nerve, and ascend to the pelvic bone, where they enter the carotid sheath that connects the outer and inner carotid arterial arteries. They then go through the carotid artery. Afferent fibers of the Vagus nerve are situated both in the lower ganglions of the Vagus nerve (nodose ganglia).

Right Vagus nerve connects to the laryngeal nerve that is centered about the subclavian right arterial and then ascends into the neck between esophagus and trachea. Right Vagus nerve passes through the anterior section of the right subclavian arterial and runs through the most solid vena cava, and then it descends behind the correct principal bronchus and plays a role in the pulmonary, heart and esophageal and esophageal plexus. It is caught by the trunk in the receding area of the esophagus, and then enters the diaphragm via the esophagus.

It is located on the left Vagus nerve enters the thorax, between the common carotid artery of the left as well as the subclavian arterial and is positioned on the arch of the aortic. This causes the left recurrent laryngeal artery upwards by rotating around the arch of the aortic to just to the right of the artery, and it ascends between the trachea as well as the esophagus. It is the left Vagus nerve then departs from the thoracic heart branches and enters the pulmonary plexus, then continues through the esophageal plexus, and then enters the abdomen. the anterior vagal trunk within the esophageal hiatus that forms part of the diaphragm.

Vagus nerve components contain motor parasympathetic nerve fibers from the various organs (except the adrenal gland) through the underside of the neck up to an upper stage in the transverse colon. The Vagus nerve is also responsible for controlling certain muscles of the skeletal, which include:

* cricothyroid muscle

* muscle of the salpingopharyngeus

* palatoglossus muscle

* levator veli palatini muscle

* palatopharyngeus muscle

* inferior, center and superior Pharyngeal Ligaments

Muscles of the larynx, also called speech muscles

The capability to Vagus nerve Vagus nerves is to regulate the heart rate of the coronary artery as well as gastrointestinal peristalsis and sweating and many other muscles movements in the mouth, which are accompanied by the sound of speech (via the recurrent laryngeal neuron). Furthermore, there are Afferent fibers that make up an inner (canal) part of the outer ear (via the Auricular branch, which is also known as the Alderman's nerve) as well as a part that connects the meninges.

There are Vagus nerve fibers which affect the pharynx as well as the posterior portion of the throat is that are responsible to trigger the gag reflex. Thus, 5-HT3 receptor-mediated Afferent Vagus stimulation of the intestine caused by gastroenteritis is the goal of vomiting. The stimulation on the Vagus nerve could trigger an vasovagal response such as that within the cervical uterus (in certain surgical procedures).

The Vagus nerve also plays an important role in the satiety response following eating. Knocking on Vagus nerve receptors is demonstrated in the context of hyperphagia (very rapid eating).

The involvement in the Vagus nerve to control the heart refers to the parasympathetic insertion, which happens on the contralateral side of the Vagus nerve, which is connected to the thoracic ganglia. The spinal and vagal ganglion nerves are responsible for reducing the coronary heart rate. In the right Vagus department is infected by Sinoatrial Nodes. For healthy people the parasympathetic tone from these sources are in good sync in harmony with sympathetic tones. The parasympathetic hyperstimulation effects can trigger bradyarrhythmias. If the heart is hyperstimulated that left vagal branch creates an aortic heart to block conduction in the atrioventricular nexus.

A known neuroscientist has discovered the fact that nerves are able to supply chemicals known as neurotransmitters that affect receptors in the tissues targeted. In his study, he stimulated electrically the Vagus nerve in the heart of a frog and it slowed. After extracting the heart's fluid then transferring it to cardiac muscle of the second frog, but not stimulating the Vagus. Second coronary hearts slows down with no electrical stimulation. The substance that is released through Vagus nerve as Vagus nerve in the form of Vagusstoff which later became Acetylcholine. These are drugs that inhibit muscarinic nerves (anticholinergics) like atropine and Scopolamine are described as vagolytics because they block the actions on the Vagus nerve in the heart, digestive tract, and other organs. Anticholinergic medications cause a high heartbeat and can be employed for treating bradycardia.

The emotional and physiological consequences

An exaggerated stimulation in the Vagus nerve in times of emotional stress that is a parasympathetic response to a strong sympathetic anxiety response that can be triggered by stress may also trigger vasovagal syncope because of an unexpected decrease in cardiac output.

This can result in cerebral hypoperfusion . Vasovagal collapse can affect women and adolescents younger than other categories. It can lead to a temporary difficulty in controlling bladder during situations of fearful anxiety.

Studies have shown that women who experience nerve numbness may be able to experience orgasm through orgasm through the Vagus nerve. It may travel from the uterus and Cervix to the brain.

Insulin signalling triggers the adenosine triphosphate (ATP) the sensitive potassium (KATP) channels that connect to the nucleus, which reduces AgRP release. It also does this via the Vagus nerve, it reduces the production of glucose in the liver by the gluconeogenic enzymes.

Vagus Nerve Stimulation (VNS) therapy employs an implanted neurostimulator in the chest because of their being used to epilepsy patients to help control seizures. The drugs-resistant effects were identified as a treatment for clinical depression. An Non-invasive VNS therapy that stimulates an Afferent part from the Vagus nerve is currently in development and is expected to undergo tests.

Clinical trials have started with clinical trials in Antwerp, Belgium, following an important study that was published in the early part of 2011 by a group of researchers from the University of Texas using VNS to treat tonal tinnitus.They verified the effectiveness of tinnitus-suppression Mice when tone stimulation was paired to rapid pulses of stimulation to vagus nerve. Vagus nerve.

VNS may also be accomplished with a vagal technique that involves holding the breath for a short period of time and then soaking the face in cold water, sneezing or tightening the abdominal muscles tissues to create the bowel move. Patients with supraventricular tachycardia atrial fibrillation, and other diseases can be trained to perform vagal exercises (or discover other patients by themselves).

This Vagus Nerve Blocking (VBLOC) measure is similar to VNS which is only used during the daytime. In a six-month open-label study in three clinics located within Australia, Mexico and Norway, Vagus nerve blockage helped 31 overweight people lose approximately 15% from their weight. In 2008, over 300 people took part in the second test, which was conducted for more than an entire year.

Vagotomy

Vagotomy which is cutting off the Vagus nerve is an obsolete treatment for the condition known as peptic ulcer.

Vagotomy is currently being investigated as a less-invasive alternative method of weight loss in lieu that of gastric surgeries. It reduces the feeling of hunger and is usually performed by pressing stomachs of patients every time.It will result in the loss of approximately 43% excess weight loss, accompanied by eating and exercising for six months.

Vagotomy is a serious issue. is a deficiency in Vitamin B12 at a later time, maybe around 10 years. This is comparable to anemia that is pernicious. The Vagus nerve typically stimulates the parietal cells in the stomach to release acid and other factors. The nerve is responsible for absorption of the vitamin B12 through food. Vagotomy reduces the amount of vitamin B12 that is released and eventually leads to deficiencythat, when left untreated, can cause nerve degeneration and fatigue, as well as dementia, paranoia, and eventually death.

Researchers from Aarhus University Hospital have demonstrated vagotomy is a preventative measure against the development of Parkinson's disease. This suggests the disease's beginning to develop within the gastrointestinal tract before it gets to the brain via the Vagus nerve. They also provide similar evidence to support the idea that environment-related stimuli, like those that are absorbed from the intestine, with the help by the Vagus nerve could cause an adverse effect upon the reward mechanism in the substantia nerve, that can trigger Parkinson's disease.

Chagas disease

The neuropathy is spread through the parasympathetic nerves that are essential to the Vagus nerve.

Sensory neuropathy in the Vagus nerve triggers hypersensitivity of the vagal afferent nerves. This can cause Idiopathic or refractory cough.

Arnold's neural ear-cough reflex in fact, an indication of vagal sensory neuropathy. It's the cause of a persistent cough that is treated using gabapentin. The cough is caused mechanically regulating the external auditory meatus, and is caused by throat infection (laryngeal paresthesia) and cough triggered through cold temperatures or food (known as allotussia).

Etymology

Latin words Vagus literally is "wandering" (the terms vagrant, vague and divagation all have identical roots). In some instances, the left and right branches are referred to in plural, and are thus referred to as vag. The Vagus was once referred to as a pneumogastric nervous system because it is a threat to both the lungs as well as the abdomen.

The Vagus nerve was named in honor of it being a "wanderer" is similar to the vagabond who sends sensory nerves from your brain to your digestive organs. This Vagus nerve, which is the longest of the cranial nerves controls the internal nerve center as well as the parasympathetic nervous system. It also oversees a variety of vital functions, such as being the primary motor for sensory impulses to every organ within your body. New research has revealed that it can also cause remarkable effectiveness in the treatment of chronic inflammation. It also became a fascinating treatment for serious and incurable illnesses. Here are 9 facts on this powerful nerve.

1. Incorporation of Vagus Nerve

An increase in inflammation is common after suffering grieving or suffering. However, overdoses are linked to a variety of diseases and ailments, from sepsis, autoimmune conditions to Rheumatism. The Vagus nerve is a source of numerous fibers that surround all of your organs , acting like spy spies. When it signals for acute inflammation, that presence of chemical called cytokines , or tumor necrosis factor (TNF) signifies brilliance and releases anti-inflammatory neurotransmitters to regulate the body's immune system.

2. It improves your memory.

The University of Virginia investigation on mice revealed that stimulation of the Vagus nerve enhanced their memory. The process released norepinephrine in the amygdala which helps consolidate memories. The same research was also conducted in humans, indicating potential treatments for other illnesses, such as Alzheimer's disease.

3. It aids in thinking.

Acetylcholine, a neurotransmitter that is released through the Vagus nerve, signals your breathing lungs to take a breath. This is among the main reasons that Botox is often utilized as a cosmetic - could be risky, as it alters the production of acetylcholine. But, you can also increase the blood flow in your lungs by breathing abdominal or by holding your breath for a long time.

4. It's connected to your heart.

It is believed that the Vagus nerve is responsible for controlling the heart charge via electrical impulses that reach specific nerve tissues, the heart's pacemaker in the right atrium in addition to the release of acetylcholine. When you measure your heartbeat and then placing it on a graph in time, medical professionals can assess your heart rate variability or HRV. These data may reveal the range of your heart's flexibility and Vagus nerve.

5. It improves the security conditions that your body is in.

If your ever-vigilant fear of being a victim activates your an instinctive response to fight or flight and releases stress hormones adrenaline and cortisol within your body, the Vagus nerve signals the body to relax by producing Acetylcholine. The nerve fibers of the Vagus nerve reach into a myriad of organs and functions as fiber-optic cables which transmit instructions to release proteins and enzymes such as vasopressin, prolactin and oxytocin. These substances relax your. Thus, with a robust vagal response, you'll be able recover quickly following injury, stress or disease.

6. It can change your mind.

The fact that your gut utilizes the Vagus nerve as a walkie-talkie to inform your brain of what you feel through electrically-driven impulses referred to as "action potentials". The feelings you feel in your gut are real.

7. Vagus nerve syncope.

If you feel faint, or if your stomach is shaky at sight of blood or feel weak, then you're experiencing "vasovagal syncope". The body, in response to stress, triggers the Vagus nerve, which reduces your blood pressure as well as the heart's charge. In the case of acute syncope, blood flow is restricted to the brain, which causes your consciousness go away. However, most of the time all you need to do is sit down in the time to sit or lie down to alleviate the symptoms.

8 Electronic stimulation.

The use of electronic stimulation reduces inflammation and helps make it disappear. The initial stimulation for the Vagus nerve reduced inflammation to a significant extent. The results were highly efficient in mice, after which the experiment was carried out on humans and showed stunning results. Implants that stimulate the Vagus nerve using digital transplantation proved to be a significant reduction, and even remission in rheumatoid arthritis , which is a condition that has no cure and is treated regularly by toxic medications. It can trigger hemorrhagic shock as well as other serious inflammatory syndromes.

9. Vagus Nerve stimulation is a brand new area of medicine.

Experts have recognized it because of a variety of research studies that have demonstrated the effectiveness using vagal stimulation in the treatment of epilepsy and inflammation. It is believed as the next frontier in medicine . Implants that transmit electrical impulses to a variety of physical structures, researchers and doctors are hoping to combat the illness using fewer medicines

What is the reason why the Vagus nerve so important? What is it as well as how do we utilize this information to tap into the health potential of our bodies to unleash our inherent healing capabilities? I've observed that there are missing pieces to not pay focus on healing. Restoring Vagus nerve's function can be to our disadvantage and is a part of every illness, no matter if it's for children or any adult.

It is believed that the Vagus nerve happens to be one of the major nerves that are located in our body, and is considered to be the nerve's heart. system. The term Vagus is derived from the word"wandering" since it is connected to many different organs and tissues and can be described as the superhighway connecting the body to the brain. It's also known as the 10th nerve in the cranial system. This is a large as part of the traditional osteopathic as well as chiropractic understandings already.

It's a crucial nerve in our system and for the majority of people, it's affected by dysfunction. It's the Vagus nerve has the longest length and the most complicated among the 12 pairs of nerves. They originate from the brain via our neck. From there it relays information from the brain's surface to organs and tissues throughout the body.

It is believed that the Vagus nerve represents the most apparent physical representation of brain and the body. This is the place where we gain this knowledge of the mind and body being interconnected, and it physically takes place by way of the Vagus nerve. It's also bidirectional, meaning that information is sent out, and information is received through the social network of this Vagus nerve superhighway that connects our stomach and all of our major organs to the brain's function.

There is a Vagus nerve makes up the parasympathetic nervous systems. I'll discuss these briefly to give you the most complete knowledge of its function and health that helps us in eradicating the signs of. We must be in the parasympathetic nervous system to heal and for optimal health to be attained. In reality, the majority of us aren't and are living in its opposite limb which is the sympathetic nervous system.

What happens when the Vagus Nerve Influences Other Organs

Let's look at what the Vagus nerve influences different areas of our body and the organs we have.

Heart

The heart is affected as a result of slowing the heart rate and increasing your vascular tone.

The Liver

The liver is a target for this. It regulates insulin production and glucose homeostasis within the liver, which is crucial. We are aware that blood sugar imbalance is among the most well-known and poorly taken care of elements of health which causes further disease.

The Gut

The gut is affected as it increases gastric juices, intestinal motility and stomach capacity. This is among the major factors driving gut health. When we're discussing gut healing that is extremely topical in the present it is imperative to consider these factors, including the bidirectional nature as well as the Vagus nerve's impact on the health of our gut.

The Immune system

This is also a factor that interacts with the immune system. It reduces inflammation which is an immune reaction mediated by the anti-inflammatory cholinergic pathway. This is incredibly important to comprehend.

The Brain

It also affects our brain and it is connected to it, so it can help keep depression and anxiety at lower levels. The Vagus nerve blocks our sympathetic reaction to stress. We'll get into more detail about this shortly.

Vagus nerve is crucial for swallowing. Vagus nerve also increases the mouth and sips information that is sent out through the three nerves in the cranial area one of which is called the Vagus nerve. It is essential for everything to be related to throat function such as swallowing, coughing, or even for your gag reflex. It also influences blood vessels, reduces tone of the vascular system, and decreases blood pressure.

Chapter 4: The Basics Of Polyvagal Theory

So far in my book, I've described the vagus nerve being a nerve that is able to help to calm you during moments of calm. Although this is the case but the vagus nerve actually two different nerve branches and each one has an individual and distinct reaction to the surrounding environment. The two branches are ventral vagus as well as the dorsal vagus.

Steven Porges was one of the first researchers to study the two sides of the vagus nerve to determine their functions. The theory is called The Polyvagal Theory, relating to the two branches of the vagus nervous system and their roles. In this view that the vagus nerve help to relax our body, in two distinct ways. The ventral vagus assists us to keep our minds calm when we are in safe surroundings. The dorsal vagus triggers the body to shut down (also called the condition of a "faint, freeze" or mental breakdown) in the aftermath of a trauma.

The ventral vagus connects the upper portion of the body. It's our social interaction center. When this part of vagus nerve activated, our brains are able to connect with other people. It helps us stay in a relaxed state and ready to be connected the people in our group. I do not use the term "tribe" lightly. I'm not only referring to your close friends and our entire communities. Our brains are built to function as the group, not being an individual. As a result, we observe and learn from our surroundings and can discern by their body and facial expressions language, what they are trying to convey. All of our actions help create our tribe and connection to it or our disconnection from it. The ventral vagus nerve is crucial in this. It allows us to physically react to those around us , by manipulating our facial muscles to produce expressions, altering our vocal tone to calm others, as well as blocking out background noises so that we can understand our fellow human beings. When we are reading a thrilling story and can feel the swooping into our stomachs as some thing happens, that's the ventral vagus nerve. If we go to the football match and get up and cheer even when we're not physically present at the field, it's our ventral vagus nerve. When we watch a film that makes us cry it's the ventral vagus nerve. It's all about the act of engaging with a community, and with our family.

The ventral vagus nerve which is the center of calm that controls our parasympathetic nervous system reacts to the world surrounding us by analyzing social cues from people around us. If someone behaves kindly towards us or displays a calm tone, you can notice that the body relaxes, and becomes calm. If someone is agitated or loud, you could respond negatively by tightening your muscles. From tiny social cues our brains transmit messages to our ventral vagus signal us that we're in danger, or are in safe. The way someone's lips move or the position of their neck or the arched brows of theirs could be a key indicator of our security. We all do this in our sleep. When we are notified of security, the vagus nerve produces physical sensations of safety in a relaxed state and a feeling of renewal.

But, if the message we get is one of danger our body's response begins to alter. Our first reaction is to search for social interaction. Eyes will open as well as our voice changes to a more savage tone and we'll show facial expressions that indicate distress. We know that someone is about to cry or have an angry rage through the simplest movements on their faces. We usually respond by trying to soothe or calm the situation. This is our organ's social involvement system trying to seek assistance from others to soothe or calm. If there's no assistance from other people, the body's body activates our sympathetic nervous system, which shifts us into survival mode. We go into fight or flight. If this doesn't work or our body is convinced that we aren't able to escape the situation, it triggers the dorsal vagus nerve. The dorsal vagus nerve instantly places us in a freeze or a collapse.

The stimulation by the vagus dorsal nervous system causes dramatic physical changes. We are less social and unable to comprehend the emotional messages of others. The heart rate decreases and we may feel like the heart rate drops within our bodies. The visceral sensation is caused by your Dorsal Vagus Nerve. When it continues to be activated the gut, it stops digesting, and we might not be aware of the fact that we are emptying our stomachs. If people are prone to suck themselves up when they are in a state of anxiety, they do it without awareness and is triggered via the vagus dorsal nerve. The awareness of our brains shuts off when our dorsal vagus gets activated. This, in addition to fighting or fleeing, are the primary reaction that people experience when they are scared by something that is absolutely terrifying.

All of these systems may help us understand the triggers of trauma, anxiety as well as depression. If we are aware that this is the way in which the body reacts to the environment that are stressful, then we can spend the time to understand how to stimulate the ventral vagus nerve in order to return to an enlightened state and social interaction. The polyvagal theory states that in order to break out of the frozen state and to activate the ventral vagus nervous system in order to do this, we must be active in a different way. Deep breathing and exhales at a slow pace can help. A repetitive activity like throwing a ball around or playing catch aid in taking our bodies from freezing and into an euphoric state. In the coming chapters, we'll examine various challenges to our wellbeing and the best way to stimulate the ventral vagus muscles to assist us in situations where we're suffering from anxiety, trauma or depression, stress and many more.

Chapter 5: The Vagus Nerve

Function Vagus Nerve

Vagus nerves play an a significant function in the body's tasks, as we've seen before. In this section, we'll look at the specifics of each function that the vagus nerve performs as it relates to the nerve system. It is important to understand that vagus nerves are integral part of the nervous system's autonomous, and is not an autonomous entity. The functions discussed in this chapter can be accomplished when the vagus nervous system works in conjunction with other nerves in the cranium. There are two major functions of the vagus nerve: parasympathetic and sympathetic functions.

Sympathetic Functions

The sympathetic vagus nerve's functions are believed to counteract the the parasympathetic nervous system. The primary distinction between them are that sympathetic actions are performed within a conscious state, while parasympathetic functions are performed in a sub-conscious state. This implies that the parasympathetic functions of vagus nerve are believed to be activated while the body is relaxed. In contrast sympathetic functions stimulate the body to be hyperactive.

The sympathetic nerve system SNS is responsible for mediating the hormone stress response as well as neuronal functions. The nerve plays a key role in the initiation of the fight or flight response within the body. The fight or flight response is a result of hormone changes that take place when someone is anxious or is in danger. The most common hormone released during this condition is adrenaline. It is often referred as sympathoadrenal since it is dependent on adrenal glands for the production of the high levels of adrenaline.

The entire response to threats that can cause a the fight or flight response, is transmitted by the sympathetic nervous system which is relied upon by the vagus nervous. The transmission of impulses as well as hormonal actions is supported by the nerve and amplified through the release of catecholamine through the adrenal gland. As this occurs it directly affects heart's functions. For instance activation of sympathetic nerve system may result in expansion of the bronchial passages, an increase in heart rate, the constriction of blood vessels and reduced motility of the large intestines.

If the sympathetic nervous system active it is possible for the body to experience an increase or decrease in temperature. Theorists suggest it is possible that the SNS was utilized in the early life forms to help in the survival of organisms since they needed to be ready to act at any time. It has been discovered that the activity of the sympathetic nerve in humans rises in the first few minutes before waking and helps prepare a person for their daily tasks. As a person you need to discover a method of stimulating the sympathetic nerve system. If you wish to be productive and energetic in every aspect in your daily life, it's crucial to ensure the body's in good shape and ready to take on every challenge. The action of the sympathetic nervous system eliminates the feeling of fatigue and laziness. When your body's in a high-energy state, you'll feel active and energetic.

The Fight-or-Flight Response

The second significant function of the vagus nerve is to trigger the fight or flight reaction, that is in essence a component of the sympathetic nerve system. The term"fight" or "flight" was initially developed through the psychology professor Walter Cannon. According to his theory he explains that animals react to threats by releasing the sympathetic nervous system, which prepares animals to defend itself or to retreat. Numerous psychologists have examined this fight-or-flight reaction and later classified it as the initial phase of the general adaptation syndrome. This is a mechanism which regulates stress response in vertebrates as well as other animals.

Catecholamine hormones play a crucial role for preparing for fight or flight. These hormones include adrenaline and noradrenalin. These hormones facilitate the rapid action of muscles prior to an attack.

There are physical and physiological indicators that show outwardly an individual's emotional state caused by the activation of the hormones associated with fighting or fleeing. Some of the physiological reactions are:

* Increase the rate of heartbeat or lung action and in this instance the person may be seen breathing heavily or your heart beat a little.

Hot flashes and paling. In certain instances people could suffer from both.

A slowing in digestion could be experienced by some people due to a decrease in stomach and the upper intestinal function.

* Constrictions of blood vessels in the majority areas of the body could affect blood pressure and heart rate.

* The dilation of blood vessels can be observed in certain individuals.

* Blocking the activity of the glands called lacrimal, which are involved in salivation and tear production.

* Relaxation of blood could result in the soaking of your clothes in an unavoidable situation.

* Erection problems during the periods of tension.

Sometime, hearing loss can be the result. of hearing

* Can result in lost peripheral vision meaning that the patient has narrower field of vision.

In the past the"fight or flight" response was observed in a different manner than our contemporary world. In the beginning the fight responses were associated with combative and violent behaviors. In the past men's masculinity person was judged by their methods of combat. It was commonplace for people to tackle issues with combat. But, the time has changed and with them the notions of combat and flight. The ancient world was the only one to associate the flight response to a predatory situation in which the victim didn't have any other option other than to flee. This could be dangerous, like being attacked by wild animals.

The battle and flight reflex can be expressed in a variety of ways. For instance the fight response could be expressed in argumentative logic debates , while the flight response could take different types, such as the withdrawal of social interaction, silence alcohol abuse, eating too much, watching television, and many more. If you're not keen on the subject, you might not be aware of the parasympathetic actions associated with the fight and flight reaction in our modern world. People still believe that people to utilize combative tactics that were used in the past. But modern day responses are unique and require an eye for interpretation.

In addition it is crucial to recognize that females and males deal with stress in different ways. Even in the beginning the males were expected to respond to stressful circumstances by engaging in an violent fight. However it was the norm for ladies to leave the scene. This is the same to the present day world, with a more of an open-minded approach. In the present, men aren't required to be warriors or heroes in every situation. It's acceptable for a man's to leave an unsafe situation, and it's fine for women to fight and stand up.

Parasympathetic Functions

Another significant function of vagus nerves is their parasympathetic function. As mentioned earlier this role of the nerve can block those actions performed by the sympathetic nerve system. While both sympathetic and parasympathetic actions of the vagus nervous system function in tandem but they are designed to accomplish opposite functions. This is among the reasons that the vagus nerve needs to be considered a component of an autonomous system. Without a system of regulation functioning, it will be nearly unattainable for the system of nerves to operate properly. The system must function in harmony to the vagus nerve as well as the endocrine glands.

The parasympathetic nerves are crucial in stimulating various bodily functions, including sexual arousal, lacrimation digestion, salivation, urination and the defecation. The majority of these actions occur subconsciously, however, certain processes require in conscious awareness. Since most of these processes happen subconsciously, it can be difficult for the majority of people to manage these behaviors in sympathetic response situations. Parasympathetic functions that happen subconsciously, like the urination process, can be negatively affected by sympathetic responses like the fight or flight response.

Parasympathetic Nervous System PSNS generally utilizes acetylcholine as its primary transmitter. Other transmitters can be employed in the event of need, e.g., the use of cholecystokinin-based Peptides.

The Parasympathetic Nervous Systems

The parasympathetic nervous systems is a component of the autonomic nerve system. This part of the system is also dependent on vagus' nerve which is the principal sensory nerve in addition to other nerves. Like the sympathetic nervous system the parasympathetic system can't work in the absence of. The vagus nerve works as a part of the other cranial nerves in the system of autonomic nerves. The Autonomic Nervous System ANS is the central control system that coordinates the activities of all the nerves throughout the body. The parasympathetic nervous systems would be at odds with the actions from the sympathetic nervous system.

The ANS is responsible for ensuring that nerves and glands are controlled without conscious awareness. This implies that the system provides signals for stimulating actions between different glands and nerves. The ANS provides the approval for the actions to occur and is the one responsible for stimulating digestion, rest and other actions like sexual arousal, salivation defecation, urination and digestion.

The activities that are performed by the ANS are described as complementar to the actions of different branches within the nerve system. Simply put, as the parasympathetic and sympathetic nervous systems operate against one another which is why it is essential to establish regulatory mechanisms. Because of the ANS both the parasympathetic and the sympathetic systems are considered to be mutually beneficial and not as antagonistic in the same way as they would be without the regulatory mechanisms.

The sympathetic nervous response as a rapid response that assists in mobilizing systems. In contrast the parasympathetic system is a slower response system that activates slowly however, it has a greater impact when it is activated.

As we've seen the principal roles of the parasympathetic system are the ability to urinate, salivation as well as digestion and defecation. The parasympathetic part depends in large part on the vagus nervous system in carrying out these tasks. We've observed that this part that is part of our nervous system depends on Acetylcholine (ACh) neurotransmitters, and occasionally might rely on peptides like the cholecystokinin. ACh works on the nicotinic as well as muscarinic receptors. It is primarily responsible for the activation of vagus nerve to release ACh in the ganglion. It's the ACh which stimulates nicotinic receptors which triggers an action of PSNS. As you will observe the the vagus nerve is a crucial component of the activities that are performed by the PSNS and the functions that the nerve performs are crucial to your survival. It is impossible to underestimate the power of the nerve which controls your digestion, urinationand defecationand other important bodily actions.

Sensory Functions

The vagus nerve as part of the nerve system, has other functions which aren't the essential. When we look at the senses that the nerve performs, we can see its somatic function (sensation of the skin and certain muscles) and visceral functions. These functions help in the operation of the body as a whole. The auricular nerve that connects the skin to the auditory external part of the canal, as well as the outside ear, is of major importance.

The primary tasks of the vagus nervous system in the upper thorax are the Laryngopharynx that is part of the nerve that controls laryngeal speech. The most significant aspects of the nerve are felt in the larynx. These include that of controlling speech and coordination via the laryngeal nerve inside. The vagus nerve is also used as the central nerve that controls the digestive tract via the branches that terminate from the nerve. The examination of the heart via the cardiac branches shows that the vagus nerve plays a major role in determining the health of the heart, and helps stimulate the heart muscle to perform pumps. The nerve also affects the dilation and contraction of veins and arteries that are near the heart, which has an enormous impact on the overall health of the heart.

To put that into perspective it is also been discovered to play an important role in the sense of taste. Different tongue fibers and the epiglottis have been linked with the vagus nerve. But, this doesn't suggest that vagus nerve is the principal sensory nerve when is concerned with tasting. The glossopharyngeal nervous system is responsible for more than 1/3 of the taste sensations that is felt on your tongue. But, the vagus nervous system is crucial because it controls certain actions in the nervous system autonomic that help to kick-start the process of generating hormones to aid digestion of food, among other functions.

Motor Functions

One of the most significant actions performed by the vagus nervous system is motor. When it comes time to start an activity inside the muscle, and then triggering movement the vagus nerve functions to make sure that the actions occur subconsciously. For instance the vagus nerve controls the majority of muscles that are connected with the larynx and pharynx. These muscles are accountable for the activation of crucial muscle activities like swallowing and phoning. Due to vagus's active activity, you can continuously swallow saliva , without needing to think about it in a conscious manner.

The majority of the muscles in the pharynx connected to the pharyngeal branches that originate from vagus nerve. This is an excellent feature of the nerve, as it is responsible for the coordination of muscles of this region. The actions caused by the vagus includes pharyngeal muscular constriction as well as palatopharyngeal.

The vagus nerve also plays a essential in coordination of the motor functions in the larynx. This is accomplished through the repeated actions of the laryngeal nerve. As we've seen that the laryngeal nerve is one of the major vagus branches located at the neck, just before the thorax. This nerve is responsible for working with other sensory glands like thyroarytenoid, and the the posterior Enrico-arytenoid.

Alongside the pharynx as well as the larynx, the vagus nervous system is also responsible for the palatoglossus, as well as the soft palate portions that make up your tongue. These actions are significant and show how superior the vagus nerve is.

When we go into the depths of our study, we will examine different functions of the vagus nerve, and how they can be applied to everyday routine. In essence, we've concentrated on the anatomical features of the nerve until the point at which we are. Prior to moving to the next section it is essential to attempt to summarize the key points we've covered in the previous section.

The vagus nerve is a part of the brain that runs through the neck, the thorax and the lower abdomen. The vagus nerve is the 10th among the twelve cranial nerves. It is a component of the autonomic nervous system. It works in conjunction with the autonomic nervous systems.

The vagus nerve is divided into various sections that run from the neck up to the abdomen. Divers branches within the nerve carry out various functions. For instance, the laryngeal connects towards the ears and plays a crucial role in regulating the sensory functions of hearing as well as the vocal components of a person. The branches play various roles with respect to the nervous system.

The vagus nerve are controlled through the autonomic nerve system. These functions are split into parasympathetic and sympathetic. While all of their functions involve sensory input, these are in opposition to one another. While sympathetic functions cause an increase in activity, parasympathetic activities bring the body into the state of relaxation. The variations in the functions of the nerve's sensory nerve are handled by the ANS that functions as a complement. But, it's important to be aware that the nerve system doesn't completely depend on the vagus nerve in the way it is now sound in the public domain.

Chapter 6: What's The Vagus Nerve?

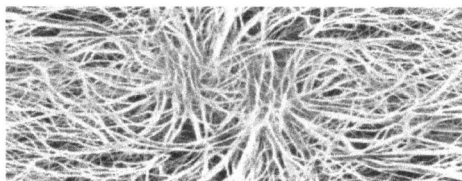

The vagus nerve is called the cranial nerve number 10 (CN X). It begins or ends in accordance with the direction of the fibers, at four nuclei in the stem of brain. They are the trigeminal nucleus as well as the nucleus tractus in solitarius, nucleus ambiguus and the dorsal motor nucleus of vagus. The vagus nerve is responsible for the metabolism of the body, referred to as homeostasis. It ensures that all internal organs function properly to ensure you are healthy and alive. It serves as an immediate link between the organs of your body and your brain. It does this by sending brain-related issues to the organs and relaying the instructions to your organs. The vagus nerve acts as the body's middle manager.

Vagus nerve is made up comprised of five distinct kinds of nerve fibres. It is described as if it were a singular but it is not; i.e., vagus nerve instead of vagus nerves. It's appropriately identified as "vagus" due to the fact that according to Latin, "vagus" means "wandering." Consider the terms vague vagabond or vagrant. This will give you a clear picture of how hard it is to pinpoint the function and structure of this nerve. Without being too specific the above mentioned points out that the nerve runs all over the upper part of the body and is the largest cranial nerve. It is a part of the section in the stem of our brain known as the medulla oblongata , which runs on both the right and left sides through holes known as the foramen jugular. Thus, there exists an left vagus nerve and the right vagus nerve that are connected across the neck and the head but take different routes when they get to the chest. In the jugular foramen vagus nerves pass between two of the ganglia. The first ganglion is known as the superior jugular Ganglion and the second is called the inferior ganglion. The vagus nerve continues to wander through the neck, starting from to the stem of your brain, through the chest, and then throughout the abdomen.

The vagus nerve is among the 12 pairs of cerebellar nerves which are all connected in the somatic (voluntary) or autonomous (involuntary) capacity. The majority of the cranial neuron only innervate the area of the head. The vagus nerve is the one that connects the neck, the head as well as the chest area and even the abdomen. The vagus nerve is classified as a mixed one as

20percent of it has Afferent fibers, which include the general somatic fibers general visceral fibers, as well as specific visceral fibers. The remainder of the 80% comprises the efferent fibers (also be aware that efferent is a term used to describe that they leave from the central nervous system) which includes general visceral fibers as well as specially visceral fibres. The vagus nerve regulates 80percent of the parasympathetic nerve systems, which means it's a major participant in our digestion and rest response. There have been a lot of fascinating studies conducted on the vagus nerve in recent times. These studies have produced some fascinating findings about how much it influences our lives and the extent to which we can influence it. This chapter will examine the parasympathetic pathways that connect to the vagus nerve. We'll also look at where they originate, and where they wander towards, and how they accomplish.

The Global Visceral Efferent Route of the Vagus Nerve

The initial kind of nerve fiber found in the vagus nerve we'll look at is the general visceral-efferent (GVE) fiber. It's the most complex. This is an apprehension nerve that originates from the dorsal nucleus of vagus on both the right and left parts of the brain stem running down each side of neck until into the chest region. It also has one minor branch on the route, known as the laryngeal nerve recurrent that is responsible for the esophagus's innervation, creating contractions that force food downwards towards the stomach. It also provides trachea with its inner part which causes the release of gas and restricts. This branch loops down the left side of the aorta, before arriving at its final destination in the larynx. The right recurrent vagus neuron can also be bent downwards. It then slips over the right subclavian artery prior to return to larynx.

The three main branches within the GVE pathway supply blood to the heart via the inferior and superior cervical nerves. The thoracic nerve splits off with the primary nerve above the Aorta. The three branches make up the cardiac plexus (a plexus is a distinct area that is innervated by various kinds of nerves). These three branches are accountable for slowing the heart's beat and reducing the force of beats and decreasing blood pressure. Right vagus nerve is the one that innervates the sinoatrial (SA) node, also known for its role as the pacemaker of your heart. The node is responsible for keeping the heart's beat constant and stable when operating normally. The number of nerves within this plexus that people refer to it as a second brain.

The GVE pathway is responsible for supplying the lungs through the pulmonary the plexus. It's responsible for the limitation and contraction of the lungs, as well as the production of mucus. If you're relaxing and resting your airways do not need to be open because breathing can be very slow and shallow. The most common misconception is Vagus nerve is responsible for the diaphragm, which is responsible for breathing. However, the reverse is actually the case. While the vagus nerve can pass through this powerful muscle, it's the diaphragm that controls it. It's the only tool that we can use to sabotage our parasympathetic nerve system. By using breathing techniques it is possible to intentionally create calm in our lives. More on this later.

The esophageal complex is the next destination to this nerve. The esophagus keeps pushing food down towards the stomach. Remember that the parasympathetic system is digest and rest. It is active and revving the digestive organs, while slowing down the pulmonary and cardiac organs.

The esophageal plexus is the next stage after which the gastric branchings innervate the stomach. They make it mix, produce digestive enzymes and churn.

The left and right vagus nerves travel in different directions at this point, and then divide into a number of branches. The right GVE pathway is from behind the esophagus and forms an anterior vagal trunk. It is the source of most celiac fibers that connects towards the pancreas kidneys, the spleen, the adrenal gland as well as the large and small intestines.

There are so many nerves within this region that it's believed to be a second brain. The organs are active to assist digestion via peristalsis as well as enzyme production. The spleen and the intestines are equally important for controlling inflammation and the immune system.

The vagus nerve of the left moves over to the side of the esophagus, and creates the anterior vagal trunk. From there, it divides into the liver the plexus. The left vagus nerve is responsible for the majority of the fibers for the hepatic plexus. It assists in stimulating glycogenesis, bile, and the gallbladder, by creating contractions to release bile. The liver is also involved in the immune system and control of inflammation.

The general Visceral Afferent Route of the Vagus Nerve

The general visceral Afferent (GVA) fibers that make up the vagus nerve comprise sensory fibres that originate from the same regions as those that were mentioned earlier within the parasympathetic GVE pathway. They are connected to the same pathway however with a different direction. The GVA fibers transmit sensations (usually discomfort, pain, or reflex-type sensations) emanating from the glands, organs, and blood vessels in the chest, abdominal and neck areas. The destination of this nerve is the nucleus oflutarius within the Medulla Oblongata. GVA fibers convey feelings of expansion and fullness from the stomach and the intestines into the brain along with feeling of hunger and emptyness. Recent studies have suggested that the microbiome within the gut use this GVA pathway to trigger cravings for certain types of foods that these populations require. The reason for this is that it is essential to ensure that you have healthy microbiome communities within your intestines more than the unhealthy ones. If you're prone to crave sugar or highly processed foods, this may be worth taking a look. The fibers also can detect inflammation. This information could be utilized in GVE GVE pathway to regulate inflammation. Inflammation, while beneficial in certain circumstances, can be extremely problematic when it is allowed to too out of hand. The response to inflammation is further discussed in Chapter 10.

There are three additional vagal pathways, however they make up the nervous system. We'll examine them in the following chapter.

Chapter 7: Activating The Vagus Nerve

With the vagus nerve becoming essential to many of our body's functions, you may be wondering what is possible to do to effectively treat the issues whenever they arise. Since it is a fact wouldn't activating your vagus nerve the most effective option when you're noticing how your ailments are linked to an inactive nerve?

It is possible to activate your vagus nerve when you need to. Vagus nerve stimulation and activation to cause it to perform a task so that you can self-regulate. If you suspect that you're feeling stressed and stressed, you can trigger this stimulation through breathing deeply. If you suspect you are angry because it is due to your inability of getting from the fight or the flight response, you could trigger the vagus nerve so as to cause your body to let go.

In essence your vagus nerve functions as a tiny, tiny button in your pocket - a switch you can switch whenever you feel you need a increase in your calm. There are methods to use vagus nerve stimulation to activate your parasympathetic nervous system, allowing you to actually end the fight-flight-freeze reaction. If you're equipped with that small switch, why not make it a point to use it? Why wouldn't anyone want to make use of the possibility of being able to actively self-regulate?

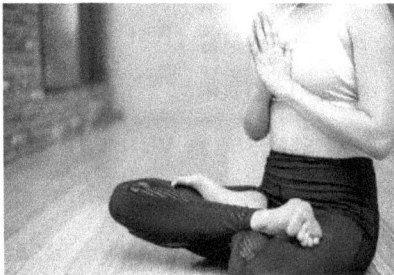

Why should you activate Vagus Nerve? Vagus Nerve?

In 1921, prompted by a vision scientist Otto Loewi tried an experiment. After a few years in attempting to discover the possibility that nerves could communicate using electrical or chemical impulses Loewi came up. He conducted vivisections on two frogs close to one another. In one case, he cut off the vagus nerve. In the second, he cut off the heart attached to nerve. Then, he stimulated the vagus nervous system of the frog that was still connected to it. He covered the heart with salinity solution while the heart rate slowed. After spreading the same solution of saline to the frog which had the nerve that was detached it was discovered the rate of heartbeat decreased. This made it clear that vagus nerve can communicate chemically with the heart and slow it down through neurotransmitters.

When the vagus nerve was activated it caused the heart rate to be reduced, but it was more than that. In addition, it shows that vagus nerves are able to influence more than the heart. If the vagus nerve was stimulated. it triggers all kinds of neurotransmitters that eventually traveled to more than only the heart. The activation of the nerve could then cause the necessary stimulation to affect every single part of the body.

This means that you are able to stimulate your vagus nerve to bring yourself down. It is possible to use the vagus nerve to affect multiple parts of your body simultaneously. The vagus nerve, and the stimulation of it is essential if you wish to address one of the many problems that arise from an issue of the vagus nerve.

How do you stimulate the Vagus Nerve

The stimulation of the vagus nerve is usually done using an instrument known as vagal nerve stimulator (VNS) device. Since it is evident that there are many advantages of activating the vagus nervous system scientists have found a method to activate the vagus nerve to activate at any time. By using an instrument designed to send a very short electrical impulse to the nerve to activate it, the vagus nerve could be stimulated.

In the 1980s, in the 1980s, VNS was identified as a treatment for epilepsy sufferers with seizures. It was implanted within the body, and connected with the vagus nerve and it is able to cut the nerve whenever it's needed. It functions like an electronic pacemaker, it transmits regular signals towards the brain. This makes it an effective device that can help alleviate epilepsy and other diseases effectively, allowing regular electrical signals to be transmitted into the brain. This makes it to ensure that people in need of the trigger can trigger it when they need to.

The device was awe-inspiring. While it didn't treat epilepsy in any way however, it allowed for the control of seizures, and in a few instances, it actually led to a reduction in seizures that people experienced. But it's quite expensive, since it involves attaching an instrument that could not work with a nerve which is created to regulate almost everything that you do to ensure your survival.

Vagus nerve stimulation at home

There is always the option of vagal nerve stimulation in your home with different methods. You can stimulate the vagus nerve at home with a variety of techniques, from taking deep breaths , singing and even trying to use the coffee enema. Whatever method you select, you will reap the main benefit of performing it at home instead of implanting a device It's not invasive.

If you are able to activate your vagus nerve your home, you are able to develop many different techniques that you can use to trigger your nerve, without anyone else around you even knowing. Even taking a deep breath is a way to do it discreetly and without anyone else being aware that you are trying to trigger the use of your nerve. If you can do this, you will let yourself be a life-saver. If you're experiencing panic attacks, you could breathe to increase the vagus nerve. If you frequently suffer from inflammation or other issues that cause inflammation then you should be able to utilize these strategies to safeguard yourself well.

In the end, while reading through the subsequent chapters, you'll discover how exactly to trigger your vagus nerve across many different situations and settings. By doing this you'll build an arsenal of strategies which will be extremely beneficial to you.

What can you treat with Vagus Nerve Activity?

The vagus nerve runs all over the body. due to that it can affect the entire area of the body as well. Particularly, it runs through the neck, down abdominal space, then then branches out to connect with other nerves of the peripheral nervous system. It is able to reach all the way to the colon and as it does, the theory is that around 90 percent of the body's sensory nerves--nerves designed to transmit signals from your body to the brain - will touch the vagus nerve, and utilize vagus nerve to transfer information.

While doing so it makes a number of important stops. In actuality, it is able to directly connect with areas that are related to:

The heart The heart: At this point, we've already highlighted how vagus nerve connects with the heart. It is vital to slow the heart in the aftermath of an event that activates the sympathetic nerve system. Vagus nerves release acetylcholine which is responsible for slowing down of the heartbeat and the decrease in blood pressure.

The lung The lungs vagus nerves also interact with the lung. Because the lungs and the heart are so tightly interwoven and interconnected, it's only natural that they will directly affect one another. Vagus nerves are involved in constricting bronchi inside the lungs. This causes breathing to become more difficult.

The digestive system The vagus nerve makes it throughout the digestive system too. Remember that the parasympathetic nervous system, which the vagus nerve regulates is located in digestion and rest mode. It is a fact that vagus nervous system must be constantly active in order to be able to properly digest. If it is not stimulated properly this can result in many digestive problems.

Inflammation: It is interesting to note that the vagus nerve is associated with the response that is meant to control inflammation. If you are injured in your body or trying to fight against infection, it triggers inflammation. The vagus nerve is required to transmit the message that an injury demands inflammation, so the spleen could initiate an inflamatory response. The vagus nerve also plays a role in cancelling this response, telling the brain to cease the inflammation.

Relaxation Vagus nerve regulates your ability to relax. By releasing Acetylcholine that activates the parasympathetic nervous system vagus nerves also trigger the activation of the relaxation response. It also has the capability of activating vasopressin, oxytocin and prolactin, all of which are connected to the reproductive and reward systems.

Memories Vagus nerve function in a way that is not optimally could result in the body struggling to create memories in the correct way. By stimulating the vagus nervous system the release of norepinephrine occurs into the amygdala. This is the brain's part which helps in memory storage.

Chapter 8: The Exchange Between Psychological And Emotional State Of Being

Presently, the mental state of our society isn't positively. There is a constant increase in depression, anxiety and stress. Even more troubling is the fact that psychological stress is being felt by the younger age groups, such as teenagers and even infants. Numerous factors are responsible for the increase in destabilization of the emotional and mental but it could possibly be due to misinformation about the human beings, misdiagnosed medications for emotional issues, an increase in social isolation and loneliness levels, a constantly shifting society and fast-paced life styles.

The most challenging aspect of all this is the confusion that people experience about the fundamental premise of negative emotions, and the absence of "training" on how to handle these emotions. It's not just about identifying negative emotions however, it is also about knowing how to respond to the emotions that are present while processing the message they send. This chapter is for the purpose of defining emotions. provide a structure for putting these emotions into a matrix of consciousness. define the process of abnormal processing and adaptive emotional processing, as well as suggestions on how to become more adaptable to the changing world.

Emotions

The emotion system is a part within the "core awareness" system, also known as"the experience system. There are three broad areas of the experiential system all of them centered on what is known as the "theater" of experiences, that ultimately determines your behaviour. The first one is how you see the world through your senses. For instance, you can witness a home or hear a car's horn and taste popcorn. This is the second thing that drives you. For instance, if you realize that it is "bad," you instinctively desire to stay clear of it. If, on the other hand, you know the item is "good," you want it , or more of it. The last area is your feelings. They are created in response to driving factors and experiences. Your emotions are intended to motivate you and help allow you to cope with the circumstances. Consider, for instance, the cat who is looking for a mouse. While it is hunting, it experiences the sensation of being in awe when it is smelt by dogs around. This causes a driver to "avoid" the dog as the smell is "bad" for cats. The cat is likely to stop freezing to keep the danger from being noticed by them. Likewise, when it senses that there isn't any immediate threat then it will go to a new area away from the dog's scent. If the cat no longer is aware of the presence of the dog, the fear that it felt will vanish. This illustration shows the process by which fear caused the cat to be hesitant to face the dog. The emotions are tied to some thing, making it a reaction "set." If you change your objectives or needs or you notice an alteration that triggers your emotions.

There are, of course, individual differences. The temperament and the emotional response can differ greatly according to the person. Certain people, and animals, are more sensitive response to emotional triggers that can trigger an intense reaction or having a difficult time trying to "calm down" after being provoked. This is the reason why a particular situation is always a trigger that sets someone "off," while the similar situation does not be a problem for someone other.

However, even though emotions are something that all of us face and deal to, not everyone knows how to deal with their significance. The education system currently within the United States does not offer an established curriculum for emotional and mental health. But emotions are something that all adults need to be well-informed about. The problem is that human consciousness is a an intricate and complex aspect of your daily life. If human brains were as mice's brains do for instance, then the first section of this chapter should be enough. But there is another aspect of human mind that mice do not seem to possess, self-consciousness. This makes the situation a way more complicated! Self-consciousness is a reaction to events that are experienced. For example, when a cat experiences fear it just fears and responds in a natural way. When a human experiences anxiety, they first be aware of the fear and form a judgement on the feeling. Humans also have the option of deciding whether or not they would like to acknowledge the feeling and then adjust the amount or little they are feeling of it. Additionally, when a cat is scared and is not concerned about whether others within its vicinity can sense that the fear. They don't even observe other animals or cats who are around them, watching their reactions towards their fears. Humans can. This is known as"the "public Self-Consciousness System." Humans are able to be aware that others are able to see their reaction to a situation when they exhibit reactions. Additionally, they can consider how others react to their emotional responses. Humans are a part of several "streams" in your mind that enable you to deal with various emotions. This can be very confusing and contradicting.

Consider an example about how a parent might react to a child's hurt. When a child has been crying or expressing their emotions in response to a particular circumstance, the parent has the option to decide to respond to the incident with either support or dismissal of their expression of emotion. This sets the stage for the way that the child expresses their feelings later on. When the child develops and develops, it determines the way that child "judges" their emotions and feelings as they grow older. This can also be a great illustration of the three types of human consciousness: the personal self, the experiential self, and the public self. This is how you present yourself to others, while you are the individual self. It is where you internalize your judgment or describe your emotions. Thirdly, the experiential self is your home of your most intimate emotions. The connection between all the three is complex and powerful.

Maladaptive and adaptive

After you've got the fundamental knowledge of how your mind operates, you are now able to investigate the experience of emotions. This is the reason why certain persons "process" and "handle" emotional states in one method over the other. Certain kinds of processing are productive as well as "good" for your health, but there are different "coping strategies" for emotional issues which aren't as beneficial. These "other" methods are referred to as "maladaptive." For the above example of the reaction of an adult to an emotionally triggered child, there may be a discord between the display of emotion in public and the inner self as well as the core emotions. If you view you or someone else because of an "negative" emotional state, it is likely to cause conflicts. The conflict could be intrapsychically or inside yourself as well as with other people or with another person who judges you.

Important to keep in mind it is not the case that all negative reactions towards negative feelings are harmful. Sometimes , there are valid reasons to experience a negative reaction or a response to "bad" emotions. The basic reaction of emotions triggers actions in a person. For instance, if you feel embarrassed, you would like to be a victim, however anger can cause you to feel the need to be punished. Fear encourages you to run away. These reactions aren't always negative. However, in the modern current world of humankind you must act with more acuity than just impulse. Your reaction to emotion should be considered in the long run and is a complicated procedure. Consider the consequences of a parent reacting to their child's emotional desires. If the parent reacted in an emotional and uncontrollable state, will their behavior help the child 20 years later in life? If all people responded in impulsive and raw ways and responses, there would be serious problems. This is why "good reason" is essential to assist you in making a your judgment about "overly emotional" reactions.

However, there's a price of limiting feelings and judging them. This can be seen by those who block or avoid, divert, or block out feelings as they arise. The fact that they aren't processing the situation is not a sign that it disappears. It is just there behind in your mind waiting to be addressed. Imagine it as "unfinished work." These feelings will inform you of important information pertaining to your objectives and/or requirements. If it hasn't completed its "job" yet in communicating this information to you, it must wait until it can.

This could be a problem when one is trying to avoid negative emotions continuously. Each day, more "unfinished work" is stored into an in-between place of the head and is waiting to be released. Furthermore, your self-consciousness system is likely to start ramping up its negative reaction within the "dialogue." You might think, "This is stupid to think this way You are foolish," or "What is wrong with you being this way?" When this happens and the dialogue is repeated repeatedly, the initial emotions are repressed. The dialogue starts to form their own inner emotions. For instance, the portion of you made of your core feelings is scrutinized and hurt in your mind by the self-conscious system. This can be a difficult and negative cycle that you are trapped in. In essence, your mind is turning on itself. This can lead to depression.

Remember how people manage their emotional systems at the beginning of this chapter. Individuals do not respond in the same manner to situations that are negative. Certain people have more sensitivity than other. This is known as "trait neuroticism." If someone has high levels of trait neuroticism, they'll likely have a difficult time overcoming these difficulties. It is because their negative emotions are more intense than those of others. This overwhelming reaction can create complicated interpersonal relationships, particularly for those who don't have a solid foundation or understanding of the information. Sadly, most do not.

Another thing to be aware of is that emotions that are suppressed aren't being processing yet. They are "lurking" within the shadows just waiting for release. This is a source of vulnerability for the person concerned, which means when something happens to trigger or release this "unfinished matter," it can trigger an uncontrollable and unexpected release. Consider people that "fly off the rails," and "erupt" emotional. Perhaps someone is suffering from an anxiety attack or even attempts suicide. They have tried to contain their negative feelings. However, after a time when they realize that the "back of your mind" becomes full when a trigger occurs, and the things that require attention are rushed up and out. Together with other stuff going on and this could result in an extremely raw and uncontrolled situation. The emotions are strong and primitive, frequently creating the situation that a person can't stop their brain from responding to the impulses of these negative emotions. A display of this emotional and impulsive reaction tends to result in more issues than solutions. However, instead of acknowledging the fact that this response was due to the dysfunctional emotional response system The person is usually even more determined to stifle their negative emotions which can only increase the problem and allowing them to experience the same response repeatedly in the future.

Based on this, you will be able to determine how to deal with emotions in a more adaptive way. The first step is to reexamine what an unadaptive process is:

Uncertain of what emotion really is.

Avoid or deny negative emotions, often coupled with criticism of the self to increase self-control

When inhibition or blockage fail, there is an overly and unpredictable emotional display can occur.

Do not revert those steps to develop an adaptable approach:

Create a positive educational environment that creates consciousness of what emotion is and how our consciousness operates

Encourage relationships and people to be alert and tuned to their emotions and how they react to information related to their personal goals and requirements.

You can regulate your impulses in a way that is healthy and associated with more intense emotions that support the longer-term goals as well as values.

The purpose of this approach is to discover the "sweet point." Let someone feel aware of emotions, and manage their emotions, and be strong and powerful. Being attentive and responsive, or adaptable is a delicate balance, but it is possible in the context of a supportive environment which is both inter- and intrapsychic to help achieve this goal.

For example, the scenario of a parent who responds to an angry child. The most common response, to discipline the child can cause problems since it fails to create an environment that is conscious of emotions and to support regulation. It can also be ineffective and punitive. This kind of behavior can result in the child internalizing their emotions, causing a problem with attunement and regulation. In contrast responding with a simple "I am sorry that you are unhappy or." is a good thing however, it is only the beginning. It assists the child in identifying their feelings and is a part of creating a positive environment. What is next must let the child learn how to control their over-active emotions. It could be a way to show that the circumstance isn't either or or, and you are not the only one to feel the circumstance (if it's actually normal). If, for instance, the child is upset due to a stubbed your toe in the seat, it is possible to be aware of the pain of pain and discomfort, and also the fact that it's not a major issue in explaining that people have swollen toes, and that it will heal within a short time. You could even give them the possibility of playing in the area, or playing the game, or offer another option that reduces the physical requirements for that particular area. This process is similar to this:

Declare that you're aware of your emotion as well as what you intended for the emotion to convey.

Provide comments that highlight the degree or importance of the situation and provide an eye on the positive. They also don't contain shame and offer suggestions for the issue that is related to the event.

A few years ago when the world was rough and life was more difficult and life was more difficult, the attitude that "suck in," was reigning. Everybody struggled and hustled to make ends meet, which meant that every person had to tackle their "problems" by themselves. This was the sort of environment who lived through those years of Great Depression and World War II lived in. However, over the past three years the standard of living has drastically changed. Nowadays, people are aware of the negative emotions we all have to deal with. There are also instances that identify negative emotions as "just" in full manifestation. This is a whole range of problems. For instance, consider instructing or coaching children. A lot of approaches shift the responsibility of a child's emotional turmoil to the teacher or coach rather than the child since no criticism is permitted. The focus is on "positive positive reinforcement." The absence of negative feedback is permitted since it could harm the child's feelings. This not only denies children of the opportunity to develop an understanding of control and attunement to their emotions as well as transmits the message that all "criticism," even constructive criticism that comes from a positive source is detrimental and harmful.

Another way to illustrate this pendulum swing in reaction in the face of negative emotion is to censor speech to avoid "offending" one. In some cases it is necessary. Like censoring the words for children or selecting words that don't negatively portray others, however in other circumstances it can be a problem. This makes the speaker accountable for someone else's negative feelings, instead of teaching people to understand and adjust their reactions to the situation. Imagine this way when you give an overview of products you sell. You say your product is "targeting" an segment of the audience. In your presentation Someone raises their hand and asks, "Please do not use the term targeting. Customers who purchase from us would find it offensive, and some are traumatized and affected by the word." The person now requesting that you take on the negative emotional reaction of other people, and not present in the room, as a result of a harmless word you chose to be used in the presenter (which can also be a frequent word in marketing and business practices).

Although people are becoming more sensitive and conscious of their feelings as well as their "good" or "bad" emotions but there is a lack of understanding about emotional responses and an absence of communication about awareness, attunement, as well as the ability to regulate all emotions, even the more negative ones. The process of educating humans about their human consciousness as well as the conflicting emotions and emotions, is crucial to the future. If you see your emotions as a signal and information sent to your brain in relation to an experience, rather than an issue you need to avoid, then you can begin to resolve issues and deal with challenging situations with much less difficulty. The most effective method to do this is through:

Inspire curiosity and an accepting attitudes towards emotions and reactions;

Let awareness and attunement be a part of your own feelings as well as those of others.

Know that the information that your emotions share is connected to the goals and requirements and then determining what it's connected to;

Recognize the fundamental nature of emotions that are typically quick-witted and impulsive, that are not always appropriate in the complex and fast-paced modern world; and

Learn to use adaptive strategies for troublesome emotions that can regulate certain aspects of the emotion to ensure it will still be in alignment with your long-term goals as well as values.

Feelings, and also the Vagus Nerve

The blood pressure drops and the heart rate slows as your Vagus nerve gets stimulated. This has been scientifically proven in all healthy and functioning people. It has also been repeatedly proven repeatedly that taking slow, deep breathing can reduce blood pressure, and cause your heart rate to decrease. The heart is an important organ with a direct impact on several other organs within your body. When your heart gets stressed out, the other organs get stressed. The same goes for other organs for the other side. when your heart is at peace and relaxed, all the organs of your body are able to become peaceful and relaxed. It also helps to relax your cells and it's that effective. When your organs and cells are at peace the body is able to send and receive messages more effectively to your brain. This will allow you to manage the emotional pendulum better.

Otto Loewi, a physiologist from Germany recognized the connection between an activated Vagus nerve as well as acetylcholine neurotransmitter. It was around the 1920's when he realized it was because the Vagus nerve sends a message to let go of this principal function, which is to relax the mind and body when under stress. One of the best and most efficient methods to trigger an increase in this chemical taking a deep breath and breathing slowly. There are many people who recommend taking an "deep breath" when they are stressed or when they seem emotionally upset. Maybe you've attempted to calm yourself by taking breathing deeply as you count to 10. But what you might not realize is that this method can actually help you auto-stimulate your Vagus nerve to release acetylcholine. This will eventually creating a calmer mental and body.

"Controlling" controlling your Vagus nerve and learning to deal with it is crucial to maintain its proper functioning. If it is over-stimulated you may experience symptoms like emotional disturbances, additional anxiety, stress and tension. Another effective tool that can be used in conjunction with deep breathing techniques to activate the Vagus nervous system is to visualize. This can result in stunning calm minds and bodies. Visualization is also a established method of calming reactions and emotions. It is possible that you have heard famous businesspeople or athletes talking about their visualization technique. They do it due to the fact that it is effective! By stimulating your Vagus nerve through your deep breathing it will help you to assist yourself in working through difficult and emotional situations.

Chapter 9: Vagus Nerve - Your Body's Communication Superhighway

The Vagus nerve is also classified as the body's Superhighway because it relays information between organs within the body as well as the brain managing the body's reactions to relaxation.

The nerve that is the largest originates from the brain, and is branched out in various directions, including the torso and neck, which is where it performs to carry sensorial information to your ear from skin, and controlling the muscles are used in speaking and swallowing, thereby in influencing your immune system.

According to Encyclopedia Britannica, the Vagus is the 10th cranial nerves, which extends straight from the brain and, despite it is referred to as a single component, it is actually an entire set of nerves that originate from the right and left part of the medulla Oblongata part of the stem inside the brain. According to Merriam Webster, the term "wandering" corresponds to the Vagus since it is the most extensively branches cranial nerve.

While it is affixed and branched throughout the body As it branches and wanders throughout the body, the Vagus nerve is the central control of the parasympathetic nerve system of the nervous system. It also provides the rest-and-digest alternative to the sympathetic nerve system's fight or flight reaction.

If the body is in no stress and there is no stress, the Vagus nerve will send an active command to slow the rate of heartbeat, and consequently increase digestion. If a person is under stress the control shifts into the sympathetic nerve and yield a positive result.

Additionally being a part of the Vagus nerve is also a source of sensory signals from internal organs and the brain giving the brain the ability to keep an eye on the organ's actions. Let's look at another vital component that is connected with the Vagus nerve.

The Brain-Gut Axis

The vast portion of the Vagus connects into your digestive system. Around 10 up to 20 percent of Vagus nerve cells communicate with the digestive system. These cells transmit a signal via the brain for muscle control that transport food through the digestive.

The motion of these muscles then controlled by a different nervous system located in the linings of the digestive system.

The remaining between 80% and 90% of neurons are responsible for transfer of sensory information from the stomach and the intestines to the brain.

The communication channel between brain cells and digestive tract is known as the brain-gut-axis. it keeps the brain updated about the condition of muscle contraction, the pace of food transit through the gut, as well as the sensation of satiety or hunger.

In a study released two years ago within the Journal of Internal Medicine, it was discovered that Vagus nerve is closely intertwined to the digestive tract, allowing stimulating the nerve which in turn, increases the severity of the symptoms of irritable bowel syndrome.

Additionally, in the past decade, several researchers have discovered that the brain-gut-axis has different counterparts, including bacteria that live inside the digestive tract. The microbiome communicates effectively with the brain through the Vagus nerve, which affects not just consumption of foods, but also the mood as well as the inflammation response.

However, it's important to note that the majority of the research did not involve humans. Most of the current research utilizes mice and rats as subjects, but not. The results, however, are truly awe-inspiring. They demonstrate that changes to the microbiome can cause changes in the brain.

Vagus Nerve Stimulation is a tool to Treat Medical Conditions

It is believed that stimulation to vagus nerve Vagus nerve has for a long time proved beneficial in treating epilepsy that hasn't responded to drugs.

Some surgeons of repute placed an electrode in the correct part of the Vagus neural nerve that runs through the neck using an implanted battery beneath the collarbone.

The electrode provides constant stimulation of the nerve which in turn decreases the intensity of stimulation, or in a rare instance, stops the excess brain activity that can cause seizures. Certain countries have approved a certain type or type of Vagus stimulation of the nerve.

For instance In Europe they opted for the Vagus nerve stimulator that doesn't need any surgical intervention.

Additional research has shown it is possible that Vagus nerve stimulation might be effective in treating psychological disorders that do not respond to medication.

The FDA is one example. It has granted approval to Vagus nerve stimulation for treatment of depression that is resistant to treatment as well as for the treatment of cluster headaches. In a study from 2008 published in the Journal of Brain Stimulation, it was found the fact that Vagus nerve stimulation can result in a reduction in symptoms in patients suffering from of anxiety disorders that are resistant to treatment, such as obsessive-compulsive disorder(OCD), post-traumatic stress disorder and obsessive-compulsive disorder.

Recently, researchers have also studied the function Vagus nerves are playing in treating chronic inflammatory diseases like diabetes, lung injury as well as rheumatoid arthritis. sepsis.

Furthermore, as the Vagus nerve is a key component of your immune system's capabilities, harm to the nerve could play an important role in autoimmune as well as other conditions.

Chapter 10: Evolution, And Dissolution

3.1 Hierarchical method of response

A development of the autonomic gives the substrates for the development of 3 adaptive stress and coping systems, each of which is linked to systems evolved during distinct phylogenetic phases. Polyvagal theory suggests that fewer social networks are employed in times of the time of danger or. The older models, although operating for a short time could cause damage in the short term for the mammals' nervous system. Thus, it is possible to experience discomfort while dealing with neurophysiological methods that are specifically designed for reptiles are difficult, e.g. Apnea bradycardia, immobilization, etc. It could be fatal for primates.

The autonomous nervous system has been hierarchically organized rather than defining the autonomic nerve structure as linear stimulation system that is based upon the sympathizing nervous system also known as a balanced system that is based around the adverse effects of parasympathetic and sympathetic pathways. As mentioned above the hierarchical structure can be identified phylogenetically and can be described as three operational subsystems that are concurrently operating:

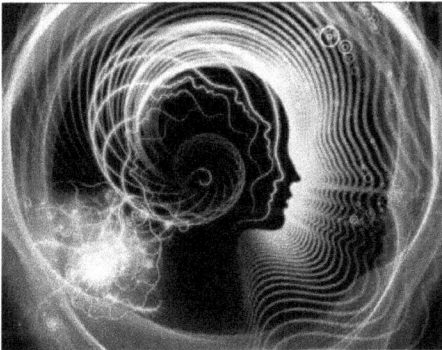

The VVC ventral vagal complex the mammalian signaling system for movement, emotion and communication.

Sympathetic nervous system: the adaptive activation mechanism that aids in the fight or flight response.

Dorsal vagal complex of DVC The vestigial immobilization system.

Each of these neural structures is linked to specific response strategies which can be observed in human. Each method is described using distinct motor output of the nervous system. These three structures accomplish specific tasks of adaptive nature to preserve and immobilize DVC metabolic resources, to mobilize to obtain SNS metabolic resources, or to indicate a low energy expenditure of VVC.

3.2 Ventral Vagal complex (VVC)

The primary efferent fiber in the VVC originates directly from nucleus unambiguus. The principal afferent VVC fibers originate in the nucleus of the trigeminal and facial nerves. The VVC is the main influence on the supradiaphragmatic visceral organs such as the pharynx, larynx as well as the esophagus, bronchi and the central. Motorways that connect through the VVC towards the organ of visceromotion e.g. The the nucleus as well as the bronchi. Somatomotor systems, e.g., Larynx and pharynx. Also, the and esophagus. They are myelinated to give precise control and speed to be able to react.

In mammals, the visceromotor fibres that connect to the heart have high levels of tonic regulation and can produce rapid changes in the tone of the heart to enable complex enhancements in metabolic performance that can meet the environmental demands. This rapid control is the hallmark of the effectiveness of the vagal brake in mammals that allows rapid activation and disconnection from the environment without activating your sympathetic nervous system. One of the most significant characteristics in the vagal brake is that the neural nerves that regulate structures of somatomotor origin are derived from branches or primitive arches of gill which have evolved into the nerves of the cranial system V VII, VII, the X and XI. Somatomotor nerves derived by these cranial nerves control the branchiomeric muscles including facial muscles chewing, arms, the pharynx, larynx and middle ear. Visceromotor efferents control salivary and lachrymal glands, as well as the bronchial and cardiac glands. The central VVC afferents originate from oral and facial afferents, which travel through the trigeminal and facial nerves as well as the visceral nerves which are located in the nucleus of NTS single tract. VVC VVC plays a role in control and alignment of swallowing, chewing and vocalization along by breathing.

3.3 What exactly is the sympathetic nervous system (SNS)

The sympathetic nervous system acts mostly an activation mechanism. It prepares the body for the onset of crisis through increasing heart rate and stimulating sweat glands to lubricate and secure the skin and prevent the digestive tract, which is a major expense for the body. It is believed that the development of the sympathetic nerve system is supported by the formation of a cluster in the spinal cord with the preganglionic sympathetic motor neuron located in the lateral portion in the spine. It has always been occupied with tension and anxiety for a long period of time. The term sympathy refers to the common understanding of this system as a nerve system that has emotions. It is compared to the parasympathetic nervous system the name used to represent an organ that is protected from emotional stress.

3.4 Dorsal Vagal Complex (DVC)

The dorsal vagal form of the DVC is primarily concerned with digestion, taste, and hypoxic reactions in mammals. It houses an NTS nucleus. NTS solitary pathway. It also contains the interuronal coordination between the NTS and the dorsal motor core of the vagus DMX. DVC efferents arise in DMX and the vagal afferents of the central vagal are absorbed by the NTS. This DVC is the main neural control of subdiaphragmatic physical body. It is a weak tonic influence on the bronchi and heart. The soft tonic effect of it is the remnant that reptiles control the vagal function the lungs and the heart. Contrary to reptiles mammals experience a greater demand for oxygen and are prone to the loss of oxygen sources.

The DVC is a source of an inhibitory signal to the sinoatrial junction of the heart via unmyelinated fibers, and thus is less tightly controlled than myelinated fibers in the VVC. Hypoxia or perceived deficiency of oxygen sources can be the primary symptoms caused by the DVC. This type of response is seen in hypoxic human foetuses. While beneficial to reptiles however, the hypoxic activation of this mechanism could be fatal to mammals. It's crucial to recognize that the DVC can have beneficial effects on humans. For the most common ailments the DVC keeps the tone of the intestines, and assists in digestion.

However, when it is controlled when it is controlled, when it is controlled, DVC can cause pathological conditions which include the formation of ulcers due to the production of excessive gastric juice and colitis. Recent research has confirmed the importance of vagal fibers without myelination within Cheng as well as Powley bradycardia in 2000. This indicates that the bradycardia's main cause could be determined by nonmyelinated vagal fibers, in conjunction along with DVC the recruitment of myelinated vagal fibers in order to maximize the vagal stimulation throughout the middle of Jones et al., 1995.

3.5 Dissolution

The Polyvagal Theory suggests a hierarchical response to environmental issues that includes the most recent changes being utilized, followed by the most fundamental last. But, the sensible approach doesn't have to be all-or-no and could necessitate a transitional mix between the the three levels of hierarchy. Both physical input and the growth of brain processes, including the HPA axis as well as the vasopressinergic as well as oxytocinergic pathways that connect the hypothalamus with the DVC are able to be established through these intermediate mixtures. In turn, this creates the neurophysiological basis of various behaviors and strategies for coping which integrate activation of several responses that are multiple phylogenetic levels. This hierarchical approach based on phylogenetics is valid as it is dissolution proposed by John Hughlings Jackson 1958.

"Higher nervous system blocks or regulates. The lower nervous system, and consequently when the higher system is suddenly disabled, the lower increases in operation."

It is believed that the Polyvagal Hypothesis of Porges, 1995 1997, 1998, seeks to destroy, not as a response to brain injury, but as an adaptive biobehavioral response to different threats, i.e., The danger to our lives. Although it is reminiscent of the Triune brain proposed by MacLean 1990 The polyvagal hypothesis highlights that a variety of fundamental phylogenetic systems have been altered in their structure and function. The phylogenetic change that affects the neuronal autonomic system is an expression of i.e. the change in the job. Structures that transmit feelings and adjust to changes in environment. Expanding an extension of the Jacksonian definition of disease and trauma breakdown and trauma breakdown, the Polyvagal Theory suggests that evolutionary responses to threats to adapt will be based on a phylogenetically-defined hierarchy. The VVC is a communication pathways and signaling allows for immediate responses to the surrounding environment. The VVC blocks the enormous stimulation of the sympathetic nerve system that is located in the heart. The withdrawal of VVC as per Jackson's theory, leads to a decrease in the heart's sympathetic regulation. In the same way, the loss in sympathetic tone can occur in the disinhibition of control in the digestive tract via DVC and the weakening of the bronchi and the core. There are a variety of medical implications of an unrestricted DVC regulation, such as defecation as a result of relaxing of the sphincter muscle and a decrease in the motility within the digestive tract. anapnea caused by constrictions of the bronchi and bradycardia as a result of an increase in the activity of the sinoatrial.

When all else fails the nervous system follows an approach that is metabolically restrictive which is advantageous to vertebrates that are primitive. For primates, this strategy could be beneficial in the short-term however, it could be deadly in the long run if it's used for a long period of time. In accordance with an understanding of the Jacksonian dissolution hypothesis, various psychologists who are identified as having affective dysfunction might be related to autonomic connections that are consistent with the three stages of phylogenetic autonomic control. The three levels don't perform any function; instead, they show control variances influenced by both visceral and oscillatory feedbacks, and increased brain function.

Chapter 11: Causes Of Vagus Nerve Damage

Diabetes

Neuropathy can result from diabetes or nerve damage throughout various parts in the human body. An extended increase in blood sugar levels in people with diabetes may alter the chemistry of nerves and cause damage to nerve-supporting blood vessels.

For those with diabetes that has affected the Vagus the gastroparesis condition can develop as a condition in which the stomach and intestine muscles can't efficiently transport food into the digestive system. When symptoms include nausea and diarrhea, heartburn, constipation, bowel constipation, anxiety and spasms there is a condition known as gastroparesis.

Alcoholism

Chronic alcohol dependence, also known by the name alcoholic neuropathy can cause nerve damage. Alcohol abuse can affect the autonomic nervous system through an effect of toxic dose that affects that of the Vagus nerve. Refraining from alcohol will repair damage to the Vagus neural damage.

Infections and complications from surgery

After lower respiratory viruses vagus nerve damage may occur. The typical signs of these conditions include nasal congestion, cough and a runny nose. There are symptoms that persist, such as cough clear throat or speech disorders, as well as vocal exhaustion in patients diagnosed as posterior vagal nerve or PVVN.

The Vagus nerve can be damaged in small or stomach surgery. Laparoscopic hemic fundoplication has been linked to injury to the Vagus nerve.

The Vagus Nerve is a part of Medical Therapy

Because of the many significant tasks performed by the vagus nerve, the medical field has been engaged for decades in the idea of medical treatment with the aid of vagus neuron stimulation or blockage of the vagus nerve.

A vagotomy operation (cutting Vagus' nerve Vagus) was an essential aspect of treating Peptic ulcer disease for a long time since it reduced the amount of peptic acid that was produced from the stomach. However, the vagotomy was not without its negative side effects, and is less frequently used since the introduction of more effective treatments.

The application of electrical stimulators (mainly modified pacemakers) to constantly stimulate the vagus nerve in order to treat different medical conditions is of immense significance. These devices (generally called Vagus stimulation devices also known as VNS devices) are extensively employed to treat patients who suffer from severe epilepsy and are drug-resistant. The VNS treatment is also utilized to treat anxiety that is refractory occasionally.

Because everything is nail when you're using an hammer, the companies who make VNS devices are examining their use for other ailments such as migraines, high blood pressure as well as fibromyalgia, tinnitus as well as weight reduction.

Additionally they are VNS applications have been shown to be promising. But, once the hysteria has been replaced by scientifically-proven clinical proof and the real benefits of VNS will be revealed.

Medical Treatments and Medical Methods for Vagus Nerve

Vagus Nerve Stimulation

An increasing body of research suggests that we are able to control and hack into the Vagus nerve system. Vagus hacks were discovered of Kevin Tracey in 1998. In his studies Tracey found that he could reduce the body's inflammation through stimulating the Vagus nerve using an electrical impulse.

It has positive effects on the treatment of ailments such as Crohn's Disease, Rheumatism, and many other inflammatory diseases. Tracey's work Tracey is the foundation of bioelectronics as a method to treat conditions such as epilepsy and anxiety. They are widely utilized.

Alongside these ailments Inflammation is also a reaction usually triggered by stress, which everyone has in their bodies. For certain people individuals, anxiety and the inflammatory response may last for a long time, leading to other health issues.

Vagus nerve stimulation is the process of placing an instrument to mimic the nerve by sending electrical impulses within the body. It is utilized to treat epilepsy or depression disorders that don't respond to other treatments.

Usually, the device is located under the chest skin which is where the wire joins it to the vagus nerve's left. When it is turned on the device transmits messages to the brain stem via the vagus nerve, and transmits the information directly to the brain. The device is usually operated through a neurologist, however frequently, a portable magnetic device is utilized by people to charge the device.

Vagus nerve stimulation has been thought to be a way to combat a number of other diseases in the near future, including Alzheimer's disease, multiple sclerosis and headaches caused by clusters.

The stimulation of the vagus nerve is an method utilized to decrease the frequency and intensity of seizures if medications are not working.

The procedure involves placing a small electrical stimulation device on the neck, close to the nerve of Vagus and also a source of power near the axis or heart. It acts as a heart-pacemaker to stimulate that left side of Vagus. It sends intermittent electrical messages to brain in a controlled manner and is also triggered manually in order to avoid the onset of a seizures.

Clinical trials have confirmed the effectiveness for Vagus neuro stimulation. Two distinct conditions are accepted for use from FDA. United States Food and Drug Administration (FDA).

Epilepsy

The FDA approved the use of Vagus nerve stimulation to treat epilepsy that is refractory in 1997.

It is a tiny electrical device that is located inside the chest of a person it is similar to the pacemaker. A small wire referred to as a lead is able to flow to the Vagus nerve in the system.

The system is placed under general anaesthesia inside the body through surgical procedures. The system then sends electric impulses to the brain through the vagus nerve on a regular basis during the day to prevent or minimize seizures.

The side effects of Vagus nerve stimulation can include:

* Sort throat

* Change in voice

* Coughing

* Breathing shortness

* Tough swallowing

* Nausea or stomach discomfort

Patients who take the medication must always consult their doctor should they experience any concerns because there could be methods to lessen or even avoid epilepsy.

Who Benefits from This Stimulation

The medication may cause more or less serious convulsions, but there isn't always any change. In all instances it is necessary for the patient to remain on anti-epileptic medications prior to adding the stimulator.

Evaluation

A physician will usually have to examine the medical condition of the patient prior to placing vagal nerve stimulators. It is essential to review the medical recordand inquire about the medical history of the patient , and the medical history that is immediate to the family members. Any information on medications that the patient has used, including electronic medications Vitamins, nutritional supplements, vitamins and herbal remedies need to be recorded. All medicines are readily available.

Procedure

In an operation that lasts about one to two hours vagal nerve stimulation can be implanted. The stimulator is connected to a nerve located in the neck via wire. The stimulator is set to be activated periodically by the nerve. The battery of the stimulator has to be replaced each 10 years. This is possible by using local anaesthesia in this simple procedure which does not require hospital stay.

The patient may experience hoarseness or tingling around the neck when pulsating. As time passes, many patients are accustomed to these symptoms.

The medical professionals are taking care to make sure that the vagal nerve stimulator works effectively and assists in controlling seizures in the patient.

The advantages of VNS could include:

* Having less severe seizures

* Having fewer seizures

* Enjoying a higher the quality of life

* It could be less medication for epilepsy.

It is possible to see that your emergency response is getting better as time passes. Six out of ten have VNS can be considered as having their numbers are halved. But, there are problems that affect about three to six percent of 100 individuals with VNS. The majority of them were related to illness and then treated through a subsequent operation.

Chapter 12: The Strength Of Your Mind And Your Healing System

It is your mind's strongest healing partner. Through your nervous system and your brain the mind sends strong messages directly to the body, which can drastically affect the efficiency the healing process. By using these methods, a sophisticated feedback system transmits precise instantaneous data from your body towards your brain. Your brain stays in close connection with your body's changing inner environment as it works alongside your body's healing system. In the words of a well-known author and physician the Dr. Andrew Weil, "Wherever nerves are, the activities of the mind may travel."

Every mental activity, conscious or subconscious is a significant influence on your body's healing and may enhance or hinder in its effectiveness. In this case, for instance when your mind is in a positive mood filled with thoughts of affection and love, caring and compassion, joy and health, happiness, peace and joy positive chemicals known as neurotransmitters or neuropeptides released by your brain could actually fill you with the positive vibe, thus boosting your healing process and improving your overall health. If your mental state is in a negative mood that is filled with negativity, pessimism, jealousy, cynicism and anger or self-criticism, revenge or guilt, shame, blame and despair, you're transmitting negative thoughts to the body through similarly powerful chemicals that could affect your healing and hamper the capacity of your body to perform its work effectively. According to Robert Eliot, M.D., "The brain writes prescriptions for the body."

If you realize how powerful your brain, and its incredible power to either work to your advantage or disadvantage, you'll spend less time or energy blameing external factors, such as rates, bad genes harmful microbes, a contaminated environment, or even other people who cause your illness, disease or lack of health. Outside forces certainly influence health issues, but in the end your health depends on the individual choices you make each and every second of every day and your ability to maximize the potential in your own mind that can help your healing process. You are the only one who is accountable for your health, which is why it is essential to be aware of this fact. As much as any force or power in the world the mind of yours can be your healing system's most experienced and dependable and reliable partner.

Mind as healer, Mind as Killer

Your mind can be used to improve your body's overall wellbeing and health, or utilize it in a manner that is detrimental to your body to harm your health. Your thoughts and your mind can trigger real changes to your body, as evidenced by the placebo effect. If you are able to train your mind to work with your body's healing system it could become your healing system's strongest allies, a faithful companion and a trusted partner. If you don't use the tools correctly, your brain and thoughts, via releases of neuropeptides that are powerful, hormones as well as electrical stimulation can cause damage to your body's health, interfer with your healing process, and lead to premature physical decline or even your final demise. If your mind isn't correctly trained and utilized your mind may be a serious risk, and become your biggest enemy, or even kill you.

Chapter 13: The Vagus Nerve

After having discussed our nervous system's parts We will now concentrate upon one of the more fascinating components of the nerve system: the vagus nervous.

If you've never heard of the nerve in question, do not be concerned. While its existence was long known but doctors and scientists did not fully understand the issue until recent. The latest research about this particular nerve led to numerous intriguing discoveries.

So, what exactly is Vagus Nerve?

The term "vagus" means Latin meaning "wanderer". It means that the vagus nervous system wanders and wanders through the body. The vagus nerve is one of the cranial ones which is found throughout the body. It is connected with the parsympathetic nerve system (PNS). This is the principal channel by that your Central Nervous System (CNS) communicates with the PNS. It is crucial in the regulation of all the vital body functions are controlled by the PNS regulates.

Since it is so vital It is a bit surprising how unnoticed this nerve is. This is the reason this section is devoted to understanding the nature of this nerve and what it can do. Additionally, we will discuss how understanding of this nerve could assist you in improving the overall health and well-being. Therefore, stay tuned as we'll be discussing a lot of details here. It is certain that you will find this informative and fascinating.

The first step is to look at two of the most important vagus nerve components that are that is the Pneumogastric Nerve as well as the Ventral Branch of the vagus nerve.

The Pneumogastric Nerve

Prior to the time that modern research on the vagus nerve began its name that it typically was given was "pneumogastric nerve". The nerve was awarded this title because the vagus nerve plays a role in the control of the lungs, heart and the digestive tract.

As the pneumogastric nervous system is accountable for the efficient functioning of the systems by the PNS. The PNS is dependent on the pneumogastric nerve in order to send the appropriate data to CNS and brain. But, considering that the pneumogastric nerve begins in the brain and makes through the lungs, the heart and the digestive tract transforms into one of the largest neural networks of the body. Naturally, when something goes wrong in the pneumogastric nerve it could cause serious problems throughout the body.

The pneumogastric nerve starts in the brain, and then exits through the medulla ovalata. Then, it flows straight across into the center of your body through the chest, neck and down into the abdomen. The pneumogastric nervous system has ramifications or branches that connect to the major organ systems discussed earlier.

First, the pneumogastric artery connects to the laryngeal nerve and then curves around subclavian arterial artery, so that it becomes visible between the trachea and esophagus. This is the place where it is capable of regulating the function of the lung. In turn, this nerve allows it to control breathing. PNS control breathing.

Then, the nerve flows down the subclavian vein into the superior Vena Cava. Then, the nerve goes through the bronchus prior to getting in the vagal trunk which traverses the diaphragm. It also connects to the carotid vein, which it is able to connect to the cardiac tissue. This is where that the pneumogastric nerve allows the PNS to join the heart.

The pneumogastric nerve is able to make its way through the esophagus, and then through the diaphragm it is now in a position to connect to the stomach. This is the reason why it allows to allow the PNS in regulating digestion.

As you can see, the pneumogastric nervous system is an extremely intricate piece of equipment that allows the PNS to control certain of the most intricate bodily functions. It is no surprise that the body wouldn't be functioning properly with out the nerve.

The pneumogastric nerve consists of the following branches that serve to communicate with the various branches of this nerve:

Anterior vagal trunk

Branchings that connect to the esophageal and esophage

Branchings that connect to the pulmonary plexus

Reflex Hering-Breuer in the alveoli

Inferior cervical heart branch

Pharyngeal nerve

Posterior vagal trunk

Recurrent laryngeal nerve

Superior cervical vagus nerve cardiac branches

Superior laryngeal nerve

Thoracic cardiac branches

They are the ones that allow the pneumogastric system to perform it's job efficiently. If the system is functioning at all cylinders communication is fluid and regulation is carried out without any trouble. If there is any disruption in communication or when the pneumogastric nerve gets altered in any way the nerve can be affected, leading to a variety of medical issues. In the future, we'll examine these issues more deeply.

It is the Ventral Branch of the Vagus Nerve

The rise of Polyvagal Theory has allowed for greater comprehension of our nervous system, and its impact on the overall health that the human body. In general, the vagus nerve is regarded as a single unit that regulates various essential biological functions. We've discussed this extensively all through our book.

In this moment, we can begin to dive into the subject matter of Porges Polyvagal's approach to understanding the effects of the vagus nerve on our body. Because the vagus nerve is located at the top of the PNS which is why it exerts an effect of relaxation on the SNS.

Let's discuss that issue more.

A person, for instance, was victimized in a small auto accident, or a fender-bender, if you prefer. The event itself is quite anxious, but it doesn't have any serious consequence. In this way, the person is simply shaken up and needs a bit of time to recover over the trauma that has occurred. In this case this scenario, the SNS was in full gear following the event of the incident as the brain was aware of a possible danger, in this case, the vehicle crash. In a more thorough examination there were no injuries, and the situation proved to be quite harmless.

If the PNS was not present then there would be no possibility to allow the SNS to shut down and the person would be in a constant state anxiety and stress. Naturally, they wouldn't be in a position to sleep or eat because of the strain placed on their bodies. This brings us back to the statement we made earlier on stress over time and its effects on the entire nervous system.

When the brain is convinced that the threat is gone The PNS starts to restore bodily functions back to normal levels. This means that the pulse and heart beat return back to normal levels, blood pressure is reduced and metabolism returns to normal functions. The theory is that all is well and the person recovers fully following a peaceful night's rest.

It is vital to stress sleeping is an amazing equalizer. This is why you will tend to be tired after an extreme increase in stress. Sleeping lets your PNS to regulate the body's processes and restore the process back to its normal. If you're not able to fall asleep, the long-lasting effects are more difficult to subdue, which can cause you to feel like you were struck by an accident.

Based on the prior scenario that was presented, the ANS was thought of as a combination of actively and passive functions. Of course, the active component is only activated whenever there is a necessity for it, while the passive part hums on the back.

This being said The Polyvagal theory suggests that there exists an additional component to the system. A component Porges identified as"social interaction" is a "social involvement" system. In a sense, it is a system that is based on the elimination of any threat that is perceived. This means that we must be able recognize whether there is a danger and when there isn't. If this happens in the first place, it's neither the "passive" aspect that is prevailing and takes over, rather, it's the social involvement aspect that is at play.

How do these three systems work conjunction?

The SNS is activated when there is a danger. Everything is in high the gears. The threat diminishes, and the brain decides that the threat has been eliminated. The social engagement system activates and warns the SNS to give an "all all" signal. So, the sole thing the SNS does is to regulate the bodily functions' parameters The SNS as well as the system for social engagement function on an off/on basis. It is worth noting that the setting that is default for your body will be active activation of the system for social engagement. The SNS is designed to be utilized only in the event of an emergency.

The ventral branch is activated in situations where the system of social interaction is under control. The ventral branch is essentially responsible for everything that happens over the diaphragm in an approach that the body can constantly regulate its reactions.

In terms of the brain, it detects the threat, but quickly erases it. The social engagement system shuts off, and it comes back quickly.

How does this function?

For instance, you're walking along the street at evening and someone approaches. You're worried that this could be a person who is threatening harm. When you are closer you realize that it's an innocent neighbor. The alarm signalled by the brain didn't last long enough to cause it to trigger the SNS social engagement mechanism to turned off in the first place and for that the SNS activated. However the brain issued a notification that it alerting the social engagement system to be in standby. In the event that this warning is genuine and the SNS would activate and the proper response would take place.

In this case, based upon the Polyvagal theory Social engagement is the primary mode of operation that the body uses. This exposes the reality it is the SNS is intended to be active only for short durations. Therefore it is possible to conclude that long-term durations of SNS activation can result in an extreme loss of overall health and energy levels of the body. Therefore, it is essential to aid the body to relax.

We will talk about this in the future this relaxing, or relaxing effect is attained through the proper stimulation to the vagal nerve. Furthermore, it's beneficial to consider the effect of this stimulation at a more general scale in terms of the relaxing and soothing all of our nervous systems, thereby helping the body achieve the proper balance between all its functions.

Another thing to be aware of is that stress over the nervous system could cause some diseases we'll be discussing in the coming chapter. This is why we like to emphasize how important it is to calm our nervous system all through the book. In this way, you'll start seeing immediate results. In reality, taking some time off from the primary sources of stress that you face You will begin to notice a rapid change in how you feel as well as the way your body reacts to numerous stimuli you encounter. Of course, we'll go into more detail about this issue when we can.

While you're at it you are in the meantime, it is advised that you conduct an evaluation of the different elements that are making you feel stressed out. It is possible that you are experiencing an issue that you are unable to control. For instance, you might have no control over your work. But, you can exert control over the methods by how you can eliminate this negative energy which could be causing stress to the system of your brain, and in particular the SNS and causing you to wander around with a strained PNS.

Conclusion

Thank you for reading through to the very end. Your commitment to this book demonstrates your desire to understand all you can about your vagus nervous system and utilize the information to your own advantage. This book was written to assist you in learning how to take care of your health and wellness by providing necessary treatment for your vagus nerve. The book will also help you discover how to manage your social life and deal with mental issues that could cause anxiety and depression.

www.ingramcontent.com/pod-product-compliance
Lightning Source LLC
Chambersburg PA
CBHW060332030426
42336CB00011B/1303